THROUGH THICK & THIN

How the Wildfire was a Wake Up Call to Transform my Life!

BY TONY BUSSEY
WITH MARK GRIFFIN

Table of Contents

I Just Want to Help!	v
1. The Fire	1
2. The Two Seat Dilemma	26
3. From Newfoundland to Fort McMurray	42
4. Packing On the Weight	80
5. What It's Like Being Clinically Obese	109
6. The Winds of Change	145
7. First Steps	183
8. Lifestyle Change	227
9. No More Excuses	260
Coaching Questions	267
About the Co-Author	271

I Just Want to Help!

It's like a dream.

I used to weigh an overwhelming 567 pounds. That weight made life miserable. I felt like a prisoner who wanted to escape my own body. I wanted to be somebody else. Not a morning went by when I didn't wake up and think that very thought. Today I am 337 pounds lighter; the equivalent of a person-and-a-half smaller. It still doesn't seem real to me. I just want to pinch myself.

Can I speak to you from my heart for a moment before I get into my story?

Let me say, first of all, that I'm not a doctor or some kind or nutritional expert and I'm not in any way knowledgeable about fitness matters.

I eat well and I walk a lot.

This is simply my story of what worked for me to change my lifestyle and the weight loss that went with that journey. If you do plan on changing your life, I would strongly recommend talking to your doctor and other knowledgeable professionals who know what is truly best for you. I only know what worked for me, how *my* life is totally different now.

Secondly, let me add that I'm not endorsing any company or, on the flip side of the coin, I'm not speaking poorly of any restaurant, organization or food, I'm just telling you honestly where I have come from and what got me to that point. They all make great products that I was out-of-control using. I still love all those foods. That was the problem. I was excessive. I realize that for me, I just *cannot* abuse these foods any more. Truth be told, I still love every one of the foods mentioned in this book, well, except for dill pickle chips maybe (more on that later), but I'm not trying to be critical of any product or business. They are not to blame. I was.

Today is a new and amazing day!

Everyday I wake up and I feel very thankful, full of energy, like I'm not imprisoned any longer. To think that I would write a book about it and be able to help and encourage others? Wow! That's totally unbelievable to me. I felt like a mess, carrying all that extra weight, feeling awful everyday, feeling like, when I went to bed, I didn't want to wake up in the morning, not wanting to face another day.

Through all of this process, the Fort McMurray fire, the change of lifestyle, the pain, the grief, the weight loss, the long process of writing my story, my one simple hope is this: if somebody can read this book and say, "here is another human being that can actually understand me, as a person, somebody who went through this, who can relate to me," *that* would mean a lot to me. If I can help somebody, anybody, if I can encourage them along life's journey, I would be thrilled.

We see plenty of big guys and big women in our daily lives; on TV, on the streets, at the mall. Like me, you probably see people of all shapes and sizes every single day, but it might never occur to most people what it's like to be that huge, what life is like being overweight. I want to get down to the nitty gritty of it, what it's like trying to put on a pair of socks (but you just can't), what it's like buying clothes, simply walking, even a short distance, or fitting in your car. I'm hoping somebody can read all of this and say, "Holy crap that's me!" I suppose that might be the beginning of getting somebody some help. I want that to happen. I want it with all of my heart.

At the end of this book I'm hoping there are those that will realize, "this guy has been through everything that I can relate to. He's a middle aged guy (or an "older gentleman"), he was *that* size, huge, but he didn't join a gym, he didn't go on a fad diet, he didn't drink any shakes or detox tea, he didn't work out, he didn't take any pills, he didn't spend any money on any special program or surgery. He just changed his life. He walked and ate healthy. That's simple! I could do that!"

It's been quite a task to write this book, but I feel it's been very important for me. I have said things and written things and realized in the interview, dictation and recording process that it's *really* hard, opening up your heart this much. I found myself saying and writing things that I had never openly shared with anyone before. There was a good measure of emotion that came to the surface. In this process I hope my transparency says something to people, men and women, but especially women who have been hurt, "there's a safe place." There are guys out there that have the same struggles, the same issues I've faced. As I share this story, I really hope to help them.

I hope I can make this as real and as honest as possible.

I say all the time, "you only get one kick at this." Life goes by very quickly. I'm already forty-three years old. I'm pretty much halfway done. I don't want anyone else to wake up near the end and realize they've wasted too much time. I might be well over half way done life's journey. There's no guarantee I'm going to make it to eighty-six. I could pass away tomorrow. I don't want to have any regrets, or anyone else to have regrets for that matter.

When the time comes that I do die, I want to look back and

say, "I've lived a good life." Life is too short, too short to be wasted on a couch, eating yourself into an early grave. There are so many beautiful things in life, wonderful people to know and magnificent places to see. Regardless of culture, race, social or family background, wealth, whatever we have in life, one thing people are always looking for is hope. There's nothing worse than feeling hopeless.

It doesn't matter if you are Muslim, Buddhist, Christian, Jewish; people just want hope. It doesn't matter if you're black, white, green, yellow, purple... purple would kind of suck. You've got to be suffering if you are purple. You need to get that purple guy some oxygen, but people just want hope and people don't seem to have very much of it these days. I hope I can share some hope in these pages.

There's a lot of people out there that are going through things right now that have feelings very similar to what I was going through three years ago. They're just feeling desperate and alone. It's not only about weight loss. It could be drugs, it could be alcohol, it could be any habit people are struggling with.

I've had people approach me in person or email me and say that I've inspired them to try to quit drinking, or quit drugs or whatever addiction they are facing. That's what it's all about for me. I think that's the power of this simple story. I had a very serious food addiction that was becoming life-threatening. If a regular guy from Newfoundland can figure out how to change things then I think anyone reading this book can figure out how to make some changes, maybe even overcome their addiction too.

I hope to give you hope. I hope you are encouraged by my story.

1

The Fire

I remember that the Winter of 2016 was the warmest, driest winter I've ever experienced in Fort McMurray, Alberta; easily the nicest I can remember in my twenty years of living there. Winters are usually *very* cold in Fort McMurray. It's common to have a cold snap for a week or more where the overnight temperatures with the wind chill reach minus thirty, minus forty degrees Celsius or worse. The city of about 70,000 residents is used to the cold. I'm originally from the "Great Northern Peninsula" of Newfoundland, Canada's most easterly province, so I feel at home with the cold.

Having a warmer winter was wonderful from a Fort McMurray perspective. Usually there's a lot of snow and ice, but consistently 2016 was fairly mild. As I would drive around Fort McMurray that winter everybody was in a good mood because quite often it was only five or ten degrees below zero and sunny. Weather-wise it was like we were just in a normal, Canadian city, with no severe, harsh winter. It was fantastic.

The Spring of 2016 was abnormally warm, not just warm, but very warm and even had many *hot* days. The leaves on the trees and blooms typically pop out in late May, but that year, flowers and trees were in full bloom in late April and early May with the warm temperatures. Everything was starting to get dry all around the region in the latter part of April. Ever since I moved to the area I remember people talking about forest fires in Northern Alberta. Fires are always a concern every Spring and into the summer. There'd usually be forest fires North or West of Fort McMurray. We'd frequently get the smoke coming into town. It smelled like a campfire right in the middle of the city at some point in the spring or summer. I remember friends saying, "Oh, yeah! We're going to have wild fires nearby this year for sure." Few expected it would hit the town, but up around Fort McMurray they'd say, "we're going to have a lot of smoke in the air this year! It's really dry. There will probably be forest fires."

I LOVE FORT MCMURRAY. It's my home and I enjoy it here. One thing I really love about the area is that we get a lot of sunshine; hot or cold, it's often sunny. If you've never lived in a forest fire affected area, let me just say that it's not good when the smoke rolls in. The air quality can become something terrible. I could go outside on a beautiful, sunny day in the Spring, without a single cloud in the sky, but there would be smoke everywhere, like smog. When you head outdoors on those days you smell it everywhere, the smell even gets on your clothes.

It would remind me of the days when people could smoke in a restaurant, where you'd step inside, and you could see a cloud, that haze of smoke near the ceiling. That's the way it often was outdoors in Northern Alberta. As you stepped outside you could see it and smell it everywhere. Springtime sunsets in 2016 were a blazing red. In late spring, the smoke-filled sunsets coming up to the longest day of the year were eerily beautiful, almost spooky in a way. Mother Nature has a way, God has a way even in the worst natural disaster, to put beauty in it.

Many people have breathing issues when the forest fire smoke gets bad. I've never had an issue, but it's definitely a big problem for folks with asthma. There were people at work who couldn't handle the smoke. They would have real problems with breathing; some days if the smoke was really, really bad, it would sting our eyes, people would need to use their puffers, some would even have to go home, just to stay indoors at home. They couldn't handle it physically because the smoke could get pretty strong.

I always felt bad for seniors and people with asthma or other breathing issues. Health-wise it was definitely a challenge. It was incredible how these huge forest fires were hundreds of kilometres away yet they would make breathing difficult in our city. In the years I had been there, the fires hadn't ever come close to Fort McMurray, not really, but blazes could always pop up anywhere. Even if there were forest fires way up north in the Northwest Territories or far west in British Columbia, we would regularly get the smoke coming our way at some point.

With the milder winter, a lot less snow was on the ground. There was not much of anything to melt off in the spring that year. We saw very little precipitation in terms of spring rains, much less than the usual. Between the melting snow and rains, it was nothing like we would usually have. The ground was dry. The forests were *very* dry. Then reports started coming of forest fires not too far away from town.

I REMEMBER those few days when it all started. We first started hearing reports about the wild fire, a forest fire that was *not* under control. It was on Sunday, May 1st, 2016. It was another beautiful, sunny day, nice, hot, hardly any clouds. I went out on my balcony and had the barbecue fired up to cook some meat on the grill. As I looked over the balcony, a few blocks from my condo, I could see smoke billowing up into the sky.

Sitting there watching the grill, I picked up my phone and went onto Facebook just to check out what people were saying about the fire, details about it and how close it was. On social media I saw different pictures from various places around town of several fires that had all started around the same time. I thought that was very strange that there were multiple fires simultaneously. Some of the fire had actually spread into city limits. As I was barbecuing I heard an unnerving sound and looked up to see a water bomber coming overhead. Shortly after that other firefighting planes and helicopters could be seen flying low to the ground to dump water.

That was pretty startling to see forest fire fighting aircraft so close to my home. I thought, "well... It's Alberta, and it's western Canada, where they've always been really good at putting out fires." I was sure they would build all the necessary barriers to keep the fire contained and away from town. I figured, it would all be dealt with and put out by tomorrow or maybe the next day.

I live in the north part of the city in a community called Timberlea. If you're not familiar with western Canada, the cities and larger towns are often broken up into "communities", not just a subdivision of fifty or a hundred homes, but often a larger neighbourhood established by several builders with a thousand or more homes. Many of the larger cities in western Canada will have dozens of planned communities of ten-, twenty- or thirty-thousand people or more, not just suburbs, but a planned, built community with their own gas stations, grocery stores, shops, schools, parks and community centres. Some communities even have man-made lakes with all kinds of activities, rental facilities, water sports, boat rentals, even clubs and restaurants. It's really cool; very different from the usual random suburban sprawl of typical North American cities. As I said, my community is called Timberlea.

The fires that were approaching Fort McMurray and even starting to spread within Fort McMurray were in the south end of town. I went to bed Sunday night, not very concerned about any of it. Then as I awoke on Monday, there were reports that the fires were starting to get worse. I started to have a feeling like, "hmmm…this is definitely unusual!"

The city was carrying on normally, seemingly confident that the professionals, the first responders and firefighters would look after it. Basically it was just another typical spring day in Northern Alberta, albeit warmer than usual with some forest fires at the south end of town.

We started to hear about "evacuation notices" where people might potentially have to leave, but I don't know if anyone was actually evacuated at that point. Again, I was naïvely confident that we would all be fine. People were getting more and more concerned Sunday and Monday, but that Tuesday, wow! That's a day I won't forget. Fort McMurray residents will *never* forget. The firefighters had been successful on Sunday, but Monday the wind shifted and the fire crept up a ravine into town and that's when things quickly escalated.

Tuesday was a day off for me. I decided in the morning that if it became available I would take an overtime shift to go to work Wednesday. I got up Tuesday morning. I looked out the window and it was another sunny day, but I remember it was very smoky; really heavy smoke all around town. I couldn't see flames anywhere, but the smoke was unusually thick near my condo.

My scheduled errand for the day was to get my winter tires taken off and have my regular tires put on. I loaded the tires into the car to drive over to a tire garage and get them switched. After that I went for a little drive out to the lake. It's a nice way to spend my last day off before heading into work. Being from Newfoundland, I love sitting by the water, just to relax for the day. My plan was to relax by the lake for a while, then come back into town, get some groceries, and get ready for work the next day.

I went to this beautiful Provincial Park, called Gregoire Lake, thirty-five kilometres (km) south of town.

Sitting at the park, I could see on the north side of the lake, a massive amount of smoke rising into the sky, right from Fort McMurray. The smoke hadn't been nearly that bad when I had left my condo a couple hours earlier.

When I had left Fort McMurray, the fires were in several spots around the city, but it seemed like they were under control. I still have a picture on my phone of the smoke in Fort McMurray that I took from the lake. I texted a friend of mine and said, "Well, I better leave and go back into the city because this seems like it's getting worse now."

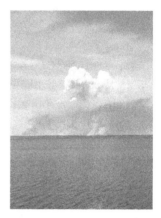

View of Fort McMurray fire from Gregoire Lake 35 km south of the city.

As I drove back into the city, I could see the municipal landfill site on fire as I passed by. It is right at the South end of town. It was very surprising to see the dump on fire. It's a very important city property and the fire was destroying it!

The smoke was billowing high into the sky, just blowing over the highway I was driving on, coming directly from the municipal landfill property. The smoke was so dense that the sky was dark as I drove past. It was like seeing a huge storm cloud turning the sky dark on every side.

I believe it was in those few hours, it seemed to me, when

the fire became massive, where it lost control, where it took on a destructive life of its own.

I suddenly hit a backlog of traffic as I drove into the south end of the city. This was about 1:00, maybe 1:30 p.m. on the Tuesday afternoon of May 3rd. It was way too early for rush hour traffic, not that we get that much traffic in Fort McMurray.

I was surprised by all the traffic because I wasn't really sure what was going on, but I could see a lot of cars out on the roads.

The highway through town was packed solid. The fire was invading the city.

Later, I realized what was happening. People were trying to get home to their houses in various parts of the city. Many people like me were in the south end

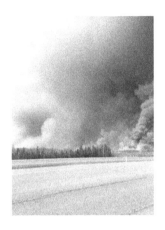

Municipal Landfill

trying to get back home in the north part of town. All that traffic was generated by everybody leaving their places of work, picking up their kids and heading home from school or running errands. The whole city was simultaneously trying to get back to their homes! People wanted to grab their family members, their pets and their belongings so they could skip town!

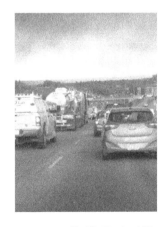

Traffic Backed Up

Normally coming in to the South end of the city, to get to the very North end of the city it might take ten or at the most fifteen minutes to travel those eight or ten kilometres. That afternoon it took me close to an hour. I wasn't really aware of how bad it was at the time because I didn't have my radio on. I was just trying to get back to my condo.

Firetrucks were having a hard time trying to get through because traffic was bumper to bumper and barely moving. The traffic was backed up all over town with people going in every direction.

In My Condo, In Denial

I finally made it back to the north end of the city, still not realizing the severity of the situation, in spite of the chaos I had witnessed. Although there was lots of smoke around the city I wasn't staying up to date on information. Initially, I never really took it all in realistically. I said to myself, "It's just a forest fire; just some smoke. It'll be out by the end of the day. If I need to get out I've got lots of time."

If I had truly understood, I would have immediately headed south to Edmonton straight from the lake; or quickly gone home and just grabbed a couple things, turned around and then headed out right away.

I went to the Tim Hortons near my condo when I got back to my neighbourhood in Timberlea. It was still open but there was hardly anybody there. After getting my coffee I came out and I didn't know what to do next. Ash had fallen on my car in that few short minutes. The fire was getting close.

Looking back on it, from what I understand now, the fire was actually consuming certain parts of the city, destroying homes at this point, at 2:00 or 3:00 o'clock in the afternoon. I was casually grabbing a take-out coffee wanting to head back to my place and relax, while the coffee shop was still open trying to serve customers who were evacuating town.

Later I found out that there was chaos in the city that afternoon. People were desperately trying to get out, to get back to their families, to collect their valuables and precious memories. I took my coffee and I went back to my condo.

I started getting texts and phone calls alerting me, "Bussey, you've got to get out."

I replied, "Get out for what?"

They insisted, "The forest fires are all around. People are leaving!"

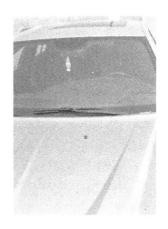

Ash on my car at Tim Hortons

I looked outside, and I could see all the traffic and commotion. I said to myself, "I'm not going anywhere. Everybody will be back tomorrow. I'm not going to sit in all this traffic." At this time, now mid-afternoon to late afternoon people were being sent home from the various work sites to evacuate the city.

Fort McMurray is an oil town, right in the middle of the Athabasca oil sands. This region contains massive deposits of bitumen, a heavy form of crude oil, mixed in with sand, clay and water. Oil is abundant here, but much more costly to extract than standard oil wells. When oil prices are high, it's very worthwhile for oil companies to extract and separate the oil, but when oil prices are low, there are lots of layoffs and Fort McMurray starts to shrink. It's boom or bust in this oil town.

In 2012, the oil sands were producing 1.8 million barrels of oil each day. The recession of 2008 took a toll on the city. As oil prices began to drop so did local production. Many projects were postponed until oil prices would bounce back again. As recovery began over the next few years the economy remained strong until 2015 when oil prices dipped again. As often happens, hundreds of people were laid off in town and real estate prices dropped quite a bit. What unfolded over these few weeks in 2016 was a significant bruise to this see-saw economy.

On the day of May 3rd, the oil companies were telling their workers to go home. There were certain areas of Fort McMurray that were burning; Abasand Heights, Beacon Hill, and parts of Timberlea ThickWood were all on fire. Homes were being destroyed in minutes by the raging wildfire. The fire that seemed mostly under control on the weekend had intensified sharply, spread into town and was now doing heavy damage.

Areas that got hit hardest by the fire were Beacon Hill, Abasand Heights and Waterways. Those three communities basically got wiped right out; burned to the ground. There were many older homes in those communities that were completely destroyed.

Even though the smoke was coming over my condo I foolishly did not understand the seriousness of the situation. I still had power, food and everything I needed to hunker down for a few days if necessary.

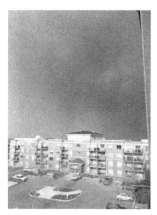

My condo surrounded by smoke.

I texted my friends back saying that I didn't really want to leave home, where was I to go?

I felt I had everything I needed, but I was being a stubborn idiot. I can be that way, very, very stubborn.

"I'm not going," I refused.

I looked outside and saw traffic still backed up, and thought, "that's not for me. I don't need to sit in traffic on my last day off before heading to work tomorrow."

People were leaving town and many of them were being pointed up North by the authorities, to the work camps north of town. They were recommending vehicles not travel south any longer because the fire was getting close to those roads. The landfill area, the south end that I had just passed through, those areas were the worst.

They were pointing town residents north at this point, north of Fort McMurray, about 45 minutes to an hour away. There are a lot of "work camps" for the oil sands workers. Most of the camps, are beautiful, almost like hotels. The oil sands companies were evacuating their workers, freeing up rooms for Fort McMurray residents, which was fantastic. I don't think anybody really knew how long this was all going to last.

I stayed in my condo. I was there, just watching TV, relaxing, figuring I was going to get a call back to go into work the next day for overtime. I figured all this would be over in a few hours or a day. I was being naïve, very unaware of how bad things were. I kept going out on my balcony to check things out, gauging the situation. I figured the parking lot was still full of vehicles, so if other people were staying, things must not be *that* bad.

Over the next while, people kept bombarding my phone, texting me. Emma, my daughter, was texting me, her mom was texting me, my family was texting me and friends would text me things like, "You have got to get out of there," but I kept refusing to leave.

I suppose a big part of the problem was that I wasn't watching the news. It was all over the TV news. Apparently it was on the radio too. I was just oblivious, I think I was watching a movie on the TV. Finally, I went out on the balcony to check the smoke again. The building manager was outside. He shouted up at me on my balcony. He said, "Tony, we've got to go."

I asked, "Why?"

He said, "There's a mandatory evacuation order. The whole city has to leave. This is law now. We've all got to go."

I simply asked, "Oh. It's that bad?"

He yelled up, "Yeah, it's *that* bad."

Then it finally hit me just how serious this was, mandatory evacuation. I said to myself, "Okay! This is real now. This is a big deal."

I hustled back in to my condo and grabbed my phone. It was lit up with texts again, so I replied to people like my daughter and a couple other friends to let them know that I was finally leaving. Some of them swore at me, and said, "It's about time you got out of there!"

I only had a minute to decide as I was getting ready to leave what I would take with me. I was watching the smoke and ash outside one moment, then a moment later I didn't know if I was ever going to see this place, my home, again. I didn't know if I was going to see my job site again or my work friends. I didn't even know if I was going to see Fort McMurray again. In those moments it fully hit me how serious this really was.

By this time it was around 6:00 p.m., 6:30 maybe. There was still a lot of daylight left but I knew I needed to get moving. I grabbed a suitcase and tossed it on the bed. In that moment I quickly answered that big question in life, "what's most important?" I grabbed some insurance papers, my wallet and I threw some clothes in. Nothing much mattered. I didn't have time to pack very much. I had to get out quickly. Being that size, around 570 pounds, I didn't have a whole lot of clothes. It was easy to pack. I took basically everything I had, three pairs of sweat pants, several t-shirts, some underwear and threw it all in my suitcase. Then I headed down to my car in the parkade.

As I was driving out of the parkade, I remembered something and I had to come back upstairs. I saw the building manager on my way and he said, "Where are you going, Tony? I told you we gotta get out of here."

I said, "I have to get something," and just kept on going.

I went back to my condo to get some of my most precious possessions. I had forgotten and left behind my most enduring treasures - handmade gifts made by my daughter. When she was little, she made me many of these little crafts, cards, notes and little gifts which were the most precious things that I own. I keep all of these trinkets in a couple of bags at home. I didn't have cupboard space to store it all, but if I ever have a larger house, I would want to have some of those little kid bits of artwork and crafty things put up on the walls or on shelves, to display the many priceless things that she has made me over the years. Emma isn't a flesh and blood relative (I will explain more later) but she's everything to me. I quickly had to gather up those little mementos before I evacuated the place for good.

I'm sentimental that way. I love things that are meaningful like those gifts. Cash value of paper, string, glue and crayon writing, 0.50 cents…family memories, "priceless." The things that Emma made and gave to me were the most valuable possessions in that condo.

I gathered those Emma memories together and quickly got out of there with the two bags. In the car I already had my suitcase. In the midst of leaving, not knowing if I'd ever come back again, I had to think in a hurry and decide what to grab or not in a second. It was sad to leave all the pictures on the walls, pictures of my family, a lot of that had to be left, because I didn't have time to grab *everything*. I had dozens of family pictures digitally stored on my phone. That's all I had for memories.

I remember after I had gathered those mementos, I looked back at the condo as I walked out the door. This was where I had lived for six years, and, at once, I realized I might not ever see it again. It was a serious, sobering moment.

It's amazing how easy it is to walk away from furniture, a big screen TV, appliances, clothes; it's all just stuff. Even the big expensive items that we work so hard to get, take months, even years to save up for or to pay off. It can all be replaced. It's just stuff. I didn't have a lot of clothes at the time, because there weren't many clothes that could fit me. I walked away from all of my furniture, a fridge, stove, some groceries, clothes, I left all of it; dishes and cutlery, the coffee maker, microwave, all of my kitchen contents. I had to just walk away.

The Slow Ride

When I finally started driving through Fort McMurray to leave town, I noticed it had almost instantly become a ghost town. Everything was shut down now. It was a mandatory evacuation for the whole city. We couldn't get gas, we couldn't get anything. We just had to get out! I might have had about half a tank of gas, probably not nearly enough to get to Edmonton.

I live right in the north end of the city, so if you keep going north on the highway, you come to the oil sands sights; off the beaten track, no major towns or cities nearby. You have to head south past the downtown of Fort McMurray to get to the nearest big city, Edmonton. Everybody was telling me to go north. Reports were saying that the authorities were recommending not to head south. The fires were close and the roads were too busy. They were making room for people to stay at the work camps north of town. I didn't want to go north. I really didn't want to stay at the work camps up in the oil sands. Once you go north, you can only go so far, and then the roads eventually end. The highway doesn't go any further, and you're right up in the middle of nowhere, just surrounded by oil sands projects.

Every logical instinct in me was to head south in spite of how busy it was and how close the fire was to the highway. So, like most Fort McMurray people I went south in spite of the recommendations to head north. I figured, the worst that can happen is the cops will be there to block the roads and turn me around to head back north. I started heading south through town, slowly across the bridge over the river, heading through downtown. It was VERY slow going. I could see the destruction, especially in the older parts of town. Smoke filled the skies overhead and the smell of it was in every breath.

In downtown Fort McMurray there's a big hill and as I was heading down it through the valley I could see the damage the fire had already done. There were still plenty of structures on fire as I drove through the city. I remember seeing this big electrical light pole right at the side of the road on fire; it seemed like something you would see in a movie, not something you would see driving through a familiar downtown area.

I could clearly see where the fire had quickly ripped through the town earlier, buildings with flames still coming out of them, smoke still pouring off of them, some with fire fighters still on scene battling blazes. I could still hear the planes and helicopters that were circling to pick up and drop water nearby, the engines labouring with the weight of water dragging them down. Sirens could be heard wailing as I drove, some police, but mostly fire trucks. In those burnt out areas the smell of waterlogged buildings, smouldering with extinguished fires had a soggy campfire smell to it, but mostly, it all just smelled like smoke. It was truly gruesome to see all of these familiar sights ravaged by the blaze, to take it all in, the smell, the sights, the sounds. I had no choice but to take it all in gradually as my car crept along as I continued driving south not much faster than a snails pace.

Heading through downtown, I mostly saw businesses burning. Leaving downtown Fort McMurray there is another big hill you have to drive up, just as you're leaving the city. At the top the hill I could see several hotels affected by fire. There was a Super 8 Hotel that was actually burning right at the time as I was driving past. I had driven past that hotel many times, a very familiar sight. To see it burning after seeing it for years as just a part of the normal landscape was very unusual, very disturbing. I could hear and see helicopters fighting the fire with those huge big water buckets underneath bombing the fires with water where ever they could. It was a disaster!

I was travelling through Fort McMurray on the four lane highway, number 63. On that day, the authorities had both north and south bound lanes turned in to south bound lanes to get everyone out of the city. Those four lanes of traffic were barely moving. That was another profound moment, realizing how huge the evacuation was. With all four lanes heading south the traffic was still barely moving.

I realized how careless I had been. I hadn't been understanding how severe the situation was, or I would have left much earlier.

A wonderful gentleman, a good friend of mine, Bobby Brown lived in Beacon Hill. I worked with him for years and was invited to his home to enjoy several dinners. As I passed by his neighbourhood it was completely on fire. It wasn't until later my worst suspicions were confirmed when I found out that entire community in the south end had been utterly and completely destroyed.

The traffic was barely inching along, maybe at five or six kilometres per hour getting out of town. Approximately 75,000 to 80,000 people were trying to leave Fort McMurray that day. It was the largest evacuation in Canadian history.

Like most places now, it's against the law to text and drive in Alberta, the law calls that "distracted driving". However, when it's a wide-scale evacuation and no one is actually driving, more like *crawling*, everyone driving was on their phone. People were texting, checking Facebook, and other social media. I was seeing pictures and videos of people's homes burning in real time; people that I knew! My city was burning down literally all around me. It was a sick feeling. I was seeing that hotel on fire. I was seeing and hearing about other buildings being totally wiped out. It seemed overwhelmingly surreal, like a nightmare.

At that time it all was very fresh, very raw. I didn't really know what was burning. I didn't know the extent of it. I was finding out throughout the evening that friends' homes were gone! The fire was just starting to come into the city at this point, so people weren't really aware of how extensive the damage was going to be. It was over the next few days after we were actually evacuated that we were finding out how destructive and extensive the damage was.

As traffic crept along outside of town it was odd to see vehicles out of fuel, pulled over at the side of the road. There were buses broken down, out of fuel that would park in the ditch, just to stay out of the way. I saw countless vehicles everywhere pulled over with their hoods up, out of gas. I could see entire families sitting at the road side, waiting with their kids. The RCMP announced on the radio that if you ran out of gas, you should pull over and put your hood up, "somebody will get to you as soon as possible," but "stay with your vehicle". They advised motorists that they should *NOT* abandon their vehicles.

Traffic was really backed up heading south towards Edmonton. I knew that there was a little village that had the nearest gas station at Wandering River, about 200 kilometres south of Fort McMurray. On any other day half a tank of fuel can easily get you there in two hours or less. With all the stop-and-go traffic it took me close to five hours before I finally got to Wandering River. It was just a sea of slow-moving vehicles as far as the eye could see.

The speed limit on highway 63 is 110 km per hour. I was lucky if I was doing thirty or forty clicks.

Some people did go north to the camps. I was fortunate to be able to get south. All along the way I was seeing more and more vehicles with their hoods up. Families parked, broken down and waiting for fuel. Everyone was listening to the radio, confused, dazed, not really knowing what was happening. We were all leaving in a hurry with everything important or of value that we owned in our back seat or the trunk of our vehicles.

No one knew if we were going to have jobs or homes to go back to, or even where we were really going to go in those early hours of that next morning. We didn't know anything. We only knew we had to evacuate. People didn't have time to plan, to check their bank account and consider the balance and wonder, "how long is this going to last?" It felt like I was part of the cast in an apocalyptic or disaster movie; it was just a lot slower moving.

I was not thinking about an insurance claim and doing the paperwork. I was not thinking about everything that was going happen over the next few weeks being on the road. I didn't know how long we were going to be evacuated. I didn't know if we were all going to be back home the next day. I was wondering where or if I was going to be able to get gas in the next couple hours. I didn't know where I was going to spend the night, if I was going to end up stuck in my car to sleep. I didn't know if I *COULD* sleep, or if the sun would come up first. I just knew I had to keep driving to get out of there. I'm sure I was having all of these thoughts and questions along with the occupants of 40,000 *other* vehicles heading south on both sides of the highway.

It was very stressful. I'll never forget it. I suppose I felt safe, but there was so much uncertainty that it was like being on a roller coaster ride in the dark, bouncing around but not being able to see; just exhausting. I had a lot of friends and family, who texted and called to check up on me.

On Facebook, there's that feature where you can mark yourself safe in case of a natural disaster or a tragedy reported on the news. I had a few friends that marked Tony Bussey as "safe." I suppose everyone was grateful to be alive and safe. I know I was thankful and very relieved.

For stretches, the speed would pick up for a few minutes at a time. I did eventually arrive at Wandering River, having travelled 200 km in five hours. I looked at my gas tank, which had even less than quarter of a tank and said to myself, "I can't keep going. I'm gonna run out of gas."

Getting Gas

As I pulled into Wandering River, there were a couple gas stations there. Both of them were open even in the middle of the night. There's a few more gas stations that they have built there since then. The huge line ups were unbelievably slow. I just got in line and stayed there. RCMP radio reports were saying that tanker trucks were coming. They said that if you were in a certain area, there was going to be a tanker truck parked at a specific location soon giving out free fuel. They wanted to get people moving. I had passed that emergency filling area quite some time ago, so I awaited my turn in Wandering River. My thinking was that if the tanker truck was filling up cars to the north of us, then there would be tanker trucks coming up to Wandering River. Eventually I would get fuel and if I ran out of gas in Wandering River, I'd be close to places with food and bathrooms. I didn't want to be stuck, alone in the middle of nowhere, so I waited there.

I sat there for about three hours just hoping to get fuel. There we were, hundreds of cars in the middle of the night, in this tiny little town in the middle of nowhere. I'll never forget it because there were many wonderful people coming up from Edmonton and other towns south of us driving up north with food. Random people were coming up in their cars, vans and trucks with gas, food and whatever they could bring to help. They were voluntarily driving a few hours up north and they knew full well they were going to get stuck in this terrible traffic going back home later. They just wanted to help. That was amazing to see.

Later we heard stories that some of these people were unemployed. With the little bit of money they had, they were filling up gas cans and coming north, two or three hours away to give it to the evacuees. It was wonderfully unbelievable.

I laugh about it now but there was a lady who knocked on my window, in the middle of the night. I felt like I was starving and she wanted to know, "Do you want a water and an apple or an orange?" At the time that's the last thing I wanted! What I wanted was a Diet Pepsi and a bag of chips and a couple of chocolate bars. At the time I was still almost 600 pounds, I was still huge. I had no desire to be eating something healthy, but I took it, and I was extremely grateful! The funny part is that now that's all I would desire to eat. I would love to have an apple, an orange and a bottle of water. I should have known that this was a sign of what was to come! It kind of *was* the apocalypse for me, at least in terms of diet.

I found out that this lady had just come up from Edmonton, 250 km in the middle of the night and she was giving out fruit and water, just voluntarily, on her own; her and hundreds of other kind people blindly rushing in to help. She was up there at her own expense and later that morning she was going to have to navigate a lot of traffic to get back home at 5:00, or 6:00 in the morning.

Even in the middle of the night it was very warm as it was almost summer. At the time, we didn't know many details about the fire, if it was contained or not. We were right in the middle of plenty of dry timber, forestry lands surrounding the highway heading south. We didn't know if the fires were going to start coming south, towards Wandering River or where the fires might go. It was a bit of a risk to drive into this area. That lady, and hundreds of people just like her were kind, generous and *brave*. Those people from Edmonton and other parts of Alberta that were making the drive to come help Fort McMurray folks, were putting themselves at risk for us, complete strangers.

After three hours of waiting to get near the pump I hoped that there would still be gas when it was my turn. Finally I was able to fill up my car at the Tempo Gas Station in Wandering River. They didn't even charge full price for the fuel. Obviously, I would have gladly paid three or four times the price, because I had no other options. They could have been gouging us, but they gave us a discount on the gas! No extra profits for themselves; no taking advantage of the desperation; everybody we came across those days was very generous! After I got my full tank of gas and headed south, traffic was still backed up.

Traffic finally cleared up when I got to Grassland, another 50 kilometres south of Wandering River. It was just normal driving after that. That's when the impact of what had just happened the last 20 hours really messed with my head. After driving all night, now it felt like a dream. It was now about 5:30 or 6:00 in the morning. I'd been up since 5:00 or 6:00 a.m. the previous morning, so, I'd been up for 24 hours. It was bright out. The sun was coming up. There was a beautiful, warm, Alberta sunrise that morning. As I was driving through that fresh smelling farmland, I remember I rolled down the window just to get some fresh air in the vehicle trying to stay alert as I headed south.

Driving in that pale morning light I thought "Twenty-four-hours ago I had a home. Now I don't know if my city's burned down or burning down. I don't know if I have a house. I don't know if I have a job to go back to. I don't know any timeline for return, if I'll ever return." I was wondering about my friends, my coworkers and my company. I didn't know if any people had been killed by the fire.

Western Hospitality

Frequently checking the news on my phone I was seeing and hearing bits of information. I was hearing about how bad it actually was. Finally arriving around 7:30 that morning I got a room at the Holiday Inn in West Edmonton. They treated me great. They asked, "Are you from Fort McMurray?"

Half awake I said, "Yeah."

They immediately discounted my room; 40% off, I think. I have to be honest. Those days were just a blur. I don't remember many details because it was all a bit traumatic, but I do remember how nice the city of Edmonton was, embracing Fort McMurray's evacuees. People were paying for our meals and lots of restaurants offered us free food.

Some evacuees fled to Edmonton. They also went to Calgary and Red Deer; I guess evacuees went wherever they had family or friends or connections; if not, then wherever they could find lodging they would settle in. I can't say enough about the good people of Edmonton and kind-hearted people from all over the province of Alberta. They treated us wonderfully well!

It was really weird to be checking into a hotel, not having any idea how many nights it would be. Mind you, they didn't ask either, but it was *definitely indefinite*. I didn't know at the time how long we were going to be evacuated. I was in contact with my daughter, and her mother and family in Red Deer. They all wanted me to come down to Red Deer, which I eventually did.

Everybody was fantastic in that entire evacuation season. My insurance company, AMA, was terrific. AMA, the Alberta

Motor Association are partners with the CAA and AAA. I couldn't believe how easy it was to work with them during this time. The first or second day in Edmonton AMA was having a big insurance session at Rexall Place. Literally thousands of people were there, it was flooded with people. I got over there early in the morning. From my understanding, a lot of the evacuees came to Edmonton, especially the first couple days, because that was the closest major city. The city went over the top to help the evacuees.

Within an hour of being at the insurance information session they had cut me a cheque for $5,000. Just like that. Boom. I didn't need any receipts. I didn't need to send anything in or fill out a hundred forms. It was just, "Here you go sir. Your policy has everything covered. Anything else we can do, please let us know." Wow.

The company I work for, Suncor, was great too; they kept paying us. I can't say enough good things about Suncor. They also communicated with us and kept us in the loop about things. I consider myself fortunate to have a great job with a company that thinks about its employees and takes care of us very well.

At both hotels where I stayed in Edmonton and Red Deer I was given a great discount on a beautiful room. When I would go to restaurants to eat, they would ask and find out I was from Fort McMurray and say, "Let us cover your meal!" That happened in several restaurants.

Already suffering a huge crisis, the evacuees didn't need to be worrying about anything more, like finances. Insurance was helpful. Suncor kept paying us. Edmonton and Red Deer spoiled us with the finest western hospitality had to offer. It was all very good under the circumstances.

Some insignificant details about Edmonton are foggy, but there are other events that are deeply etched in my memory, especially some of the details as we started hearing reports of what was happening in Fort McMurray. The fire had gotten so big that it was out of control. It was burning fast. We heard reports of the damage that had been done. We heard of certain areas of town that had been ravaged by the fire. I remember looking on Facebook to see precisely how close the fire was to my home. My home seemed to be untouched but who knew for sure?

I vividly remember getting in touch with other friends that had been evacuated. I went out for a meal with several of them. Through tears some of these friends would be telling the stories of their loss. It was painful to learn how some of them had lost their homes, their vehicles, some even lost their pets as well.

We were all so thankful, thank God, that nobody got killed directly by fire. There was one young lady, 15 years of age, and another young man that died in a traffic accident fleeing the fire, but nobody burned or suffered a smoke inhalation death. We didn't know all the details of the evacuation at the time but we were hearing that about 80,000 people left the city all at once. With fire all around us, it's absolutely amazing no one was killed by the fire.

I've seen pictures and videos afterwards of people driving through fire and smoke to get out of town coming down through Fort McMurray where the fire was only a few feet away from them. I was fortunate I didn't have to deal with driving that close to the blaze. That must have been extremely stressful. With the fire being so close to the roads and with fire being so unpredictable, what if that extreme heat had blown out tires? Again, it's a wonder no one was killed, we were all very fortunate.

It was a comfort to be in the familiar town limits of Red Deer. Emma was ten years old when her mom had first moved down to Red Deer from Fort McMurray so I had become familiar with the city after many visits. Emma and her mom had already been down there for about five years at that time, settled in well. That summer of the fire, Emma was fifteen.

AS UNSETTLING AND as painful as it was to be evacuated, I honestly believe, to this day, I would not be alive today if it were not for the wildfires that swept through Fort McMurray. I have sat through several interviews to share my story and I often say that the Fort McMurray fire saved my life and I *really* believe it. This evacuation and especially the second evacuation a couple weeks later served as a wakeup call that would change my life and my lifestyle forever.

2

The Two Seat Dilemma

After about a week in Red Deer I got called in to go back to work in the oil sands. The fires seemed to be dying down at that time. They told me they were going to fly me back to work. I hated flying.

At the time, I was almost 600 pounds. Plane travel was really awkward, trying to wedge myself into already crowded seats. Suncor had their own private planes with which they planned to fly work crews out of Edmonton. When I arrived at the airport, I parked my car in the long-term parking lot. In the terminal I approached the airline boarding desk and talked to a staff member with my special request, "I'm going to need some assistance - a seat belt extension and a seat with an empty seat beside it." All of this was very embarrassing for me. I was anxious about the whole ordeal.

The plan was to send us back up to work and lodge us at a work camp, north of Fort McMurray. No one was allowed back into Fort McMurray yet. The city was not even close to welcoming residents again. They were still managing the effects of the fire there. Long after it was under control they needed a lot of time to restore essential services like power and water. It was a huge undertaking to re-open the city.

I boarded the plane. On this flight, they had a row of two seats on one side of the aircraft and a single row with one seat along the other side of the plane by the windows. They let me board the plane first as a "special assistance" passenger. I got to the row with two seats looking for a spot. I had hoped to find what many planes have, double seats where the arm rest goes up between the seats so I would have some room. However, the armrest was fixed, unmovable, so I couldn't sit there. I was stressed about it. I was about ready to walk off the plane because of how embarrassed I felt. A mechanic friend of mine was sitting on the single seat side of the aisle. He said, "Try this one Bussey. Usually these seem a bit bigger." So I managed to squeeze into the single seat, but just barely. I had to get the seat belt extension to get it done up. A lot of these guys on the plane heading back to work had known me for years. We had all worked together. They didn't look at me any differently, so that situation wasn't as embarrassing as it could have been.

After a quick flight we got up to Firebag airport about 150 km north of Fort McMurray. We were then bussed to a work camp. My camp room was tiny with a little twin bed; fine for a normal size person, but for me, it was very tight. The bathroom was a shared. The stand up shower was so small I could barely move around to wash myself.

We were scheduled to be at the camp for nine days. I think that the company was planning to bring up some senior employees to get things up and running again before they started the regular shifts back to work. All the reports were saying that the fire seemed like it was getting under control.

We were settled into the camp. The plan was that the next day we would start back to work, getting the shop rolling again. For those nine days I was supposed to work at the shop where I normally work. My shop is about a 45-minute drive north of

Fort McMurray. The camps where we were staying that week were another 40-minute drive North of that same shop.

These work camps were almost like big hotels where they looked after us well. In the morning at the camp they'd serve a beautiful breakfast in the kitchen area and then they sent us off for the shift with packed lunches. I would take a couple of delicious entrées, snacks, desserts, whatever I wanted. We could take anything we needed for the day and return for supper in the evening, back at camp.

Every camp was different. The camp I was staying at had a lot of accommodation trailers with sleeping units all joined together. Down the hall, beyond all the rooms, there was a huge kitchen. Some camps had different facilities with workout areas, lounges, coffee bars and even play grounds for the families with kids. This particular camp was mostly just rooms and a kitchen and some lounge areas. That first night we settled in and prepared to head out the next morning after breakfast.

When we got to work that first morning there was ash falling at the work site. I remember a few hours later by noon it really started to get darker. It was completely dark like I was on night shift. There was a red glow in the distance, but smoke filled the sky. At 3:00 o'clock in the afternoon the sky was as dark as midnight. It was fine to breathe. The air smelled smokey and all the smoke was blocking out the sunlight overhead. I will never forget that as long as I live. It was very eerie with ash falling from the dark sky.

Apparently in the last 24 hours or so during that first shift back to work, the wind had shifted. It was plenty safe to fly us back to work when they did, but these wild fires don't follow a certain schedule or a travel plan. What was originally a safe zone, was starting to potentially become a threatened area.

Not wanting to take any chances, they let us finish our shift, but that was probably going to be it for work. There was a plan to evacuate us again! They told us that with the wind shifting it was quickly becoming too smoky in the area to continue working. It wasn't smoky inside the buildings at work or at the camp. We didn't open our windows. There was a lot of smoke around and of course, I could smell smoke strongly when I was outdoors, but it seemed safe.

There were rumours that the wild fire had shifted even more in the last few hours and was getting closer to the camps. Where we were working would probably be fine, but other camps, 40 minutes north of us were in possible danger. Later that evening, when our shift was done, the oncoming shift was not even brought into work. Our shift was the first and last back to work in that shop. The fire was getting closer to the various work sites, but it was especially starting to threaten some of the camps at this time. The fire continued to build and started to spread in unwanted directions. That is, after all, why they call them "wild" fires.

Imagine all the logistics involved for these oil companies with having to charter planes and buses, bringing in staff for housing and cooking, flying employees back to work, and we were only there for one shift — that second shift never even made it to work at all. For safety reasons they had to immediately make plans to evacuate everybody barely 24 hours after getting us all back to work. This was serious!

During that first shift back on the job we were hearing stories that a couple of the work camps were on fire. What some of us initially feared was that *our* camp was one of the camps that was on fire, where we all were staying. What we had heard was that one of the camps had burned right to the ground. I was thinking, "Oh no, this is NOT great. Everything I own, all my insurance papers, the little that I had is gone! My clothes and papers that I hastily packed up a few days ago leaving my condo in Fort McMurray, that stuff is, or was, all in my suitcase back at the camp! This is unbelievable." My other few things, the precious memories from Emma, thankfully, they were safely in my car back in the Edmonton airport parking lot.

We were just getting to the end of our first 12 hour shift when word came that they would definitely be evacuating us soon after we got back to the camp. Suncor was always wanting to protect their employees. When we did get on the bus to be shuttled back to camp we were told it was a *different* camp that had burned to the ground. Our camp was safe. I was relieved to know that I still had my few clothes and my insurance papers. They would get us back to camp and then the plan was to evacuate us soon.

That shift we had just finished was from 7:00 AM to 7:00 PM. Arriving back at camp we were told to be packed up and ready to go and that details would follow. All night long we weren't really sure when we were going to be evacuated. We just kept hoping to get some information, but it was quiet. We ended up being there all that night, not getting much sleep. They had to arrange the buses and then flights. They had to evacuate everybody, with priority going to the people that were closest to the danger first, then everybody else.

The next day the buses finally came. We waited around all morning as other camps were prioritized, but finally in the early afternoon, the buses rolled in for our camp; the second evacuation was on. It was stressful since every one of us had already been *emergency evacuated* once before, twelve days prior. Now we were going through it again, so we knew it was all very serious, very real.

There was still a possible element of danger about the whole thing. I don't think any of us really felt safe until after we were flown out and landed safely a few hundred kilometres away. That fire was moving really fast. It was jumping over fire breaks and still growing because the entire province was dry tinder for the blaze.

THE FIRST RESPONDERS, the fire fighters were nothing short of heroic; the hours they were putting in trying to save homes, trying to fight the fires in the city and at the camps, they sacrificed immensely to help and serve us all. Thanks to their exceptional work and all the safety protocols in place, we were fortunate enough not to have anybody get killed directly as a result of the fire. Ironically and tragically, there was one car accident where a girl and her step-cousin was killed; she was the daughter of a deputy fire chief. Emily Ryan was a 15-year old triplet who was killed in a fiery car crash fleeing the city, along with Aaron Hodgson her older relative. It's truly a miracle that over 80,000 people were evacuated between our city, other little towns and the work camps with no other fatalities. As I mentioned, it was the largest evacuation in the history of Canada.

As we stood in line waiting to be evacuated, there was a level of anxiety among the workers. The smell of smoke was strong in the air. There were huge clouds of smoke in the distance. We knew things must have been serious for them to fly us back to work and then fly us right back out again after only one shift. Safety is always a huge priority to our company. This was obviously a very serious situation.

FINALLY, the buses started rolling into our camp. I had my suitcase with my few clothes, my insurance papers and my wallet. I was ready to get out. I was near the back of the lineup waiting for the bus. As the bus rolled up a manager came along and he moved me from the back of the line up to the front for priority boarding. I'm sure they didn't want me passing out. That was humiliating!

At the time I hated being moved to the front of the line, because I didn't want or appreciate the extra attention. I hated having any attention drawn towards me at any time. Any big person you might talk to, especially people my former size will tell you the exact same thing. They don't want anybody staring at them. They just want to blend in and not have people notice them at all. I understand why they moved me to the front of the line, because the last thing anyone would want in that heat is a problem with an unmanageable big guy. I remember how hot it was. This was early May 2016, it was unusually, unseasonably hot, often into the low 30's (Celsius) those days. With that unbearable heat, they wanted to evacuate us quickly. The sooner I got on the bus, the better it would be for everyone.

For a big guy, that alone was a lot of shame for me to handle because now even more eyes were on me. All of these people that were in front of me in the line up were now behind me looking at my huge back. All these poor souls that were just wanting to get back to their families, now they had to wait a little longer because this big guy just got to the front of the line. I felt horrible. It was embarrassing and I wanted nothing more than to crawl under a rock.

I can totally understand why they did it. If I was getting on the same bus with some huge gentleman, I would have done the same thing and moved him ahead in the line-up. In desperate times, the right thing to do is prioritize the handicapped. At that season in my life, that size, I was definitely a liability to those around me.

What if the big guy had fainted in the heat? Then what would be done? Seriously. Get a forklift? Or a tractor? How could anyone lift a 600-pound guy who has passed out? Was there a stretcher or wheelchair big enough to hold me? Who was going to be able to lift up a 600-pounds of limp weight? I was a disaster waiting to happen. There's no equipment there to deal with a guy that big. The camp was not equipped for such a thing. There is no place in the world equipped to deal with a guy that big.

So the manager pulled me out of line and he got me on a bus as soon as possible, putting me at the very front of the line up. I remember the shameful feeling as I walked up the steps onto the bus ahead of all my peers. As I looked down the empty centre aisle, I just wanted to hide or run away and forget about the whole thing. The bus quickly filled up and was getting ready to leave, but there was a single seat next to me, still empty, but I was spilling uncomfortably over the armrest area into the seat beside me. In reality, I was taking up half of the empty seat.

WHEN I LOOKED out the window of the bus, I could see all these people lined up, waiting for a seat. Waiting to get to a safe place, waiting to get home, waiting to see their spouses, their kids, their loved ones, their parents. Here I am, a single guy, with no one waiting for me anywhere nearby and I am the first in that line to evacuate. I was first in line **and** taking up someone else's spot because I was so huge that I needed two seats.

THE PAINFUL MEMORY of that entire scene has played over in my head countless times. As I looked out into the parking lot I could see all those people and they're looking in at the bus to see if there are any empty seats. One of those people, one more person could have got on the bus if I was a normal size.

That's when the full impact of my selfishness first hit me like a ton of bricks. One of those people could have been home earlier. This was around 2:00 o'clock in the afternoon. It was my understanding that by the time they got more buses back there to evacuate the rest of the people, it was around 8:30 p.m., so, because of my size, somebody had to wait many hours in that disaster, in that danger zone. I know there were hundreds of people they had to get out that afternoon, but I couldn't stop thinking about the one, the one whose seat I had taken, the one I had ripped off.

That haunting thought tormented me.

THE BUSES SHUTTLED us to the airport up north of the camps. Firebag Airport is a full-service airport, 118 km northeast of Fort McMurray, not far from Firebag River which gives the airport its name. It's a nice facility, a typical small airport. They can accommodate all the small and even mid-sized commercial air carriers.

When we arrived, we were waiting on the buses. Planes were landing and as soon as they would fill up, in a matter of minutes they were reloading and taking off again. There were planes from WestJet, Air Canada, Canadian North and various charter companies. I'd never seen anything like it. I'm sure every sizeable plane in western Canada was being sent to Fort McMurray. All kinds of planes were landing, picking people up, big and medium planes, every available company, everything and anything they could do to safely and quickly get people out of there. It was all free. Our safety was the priority. There was no need to slow things down or complicate things with ticket distribution or purchases. This was an emergency! There were mostly Oil Sands workers getting out, but I think there were some Fort McMurray residents there too who had been housed at the camps from the first evacuation. Most of us in the second evacuation were predominantly workers.

We had to wait a while for all the planes to land. We waited on the bus for hours awaiting our turn. Our buses were in a big bus queue, waiting right there on the road. As I waited all this clutter was going through my mind. I kept looking down and seeing that empty seat, half seat, beside me. It had a big effect on me. With that and everything else that had been going on for the last 14 years, it was shaping up to be the final straw.

As we eventually got up to the tarmac, we evacuees finally got off the bus to see staff and emergency personnel pointing us in the right direction. Their simple question was, "Edmonton or Calgary?" That's all they asked. I chose Edmonton because my car was there in the airport parking lot and I figured I would likely head back to Red Deer again to be near my daughter Emma. They pointed me to the left and said "that plane." They asked me to show my Suncor ID, which I suppose served as my ticket, and my license, which functioned as my government issued photo ID. That was it. Knowing how many people were waiting, it was incredibly quick, safe and efficient.

I boarded a big charter plane. I don't remember the name of the charter company; it wasn't one I had heard of or flown before. It was a big, beautiful plane, I'd guess a 737 or something like that; there was a long centre aisle with 3 seats on either side of the aisle. The plane was about to be loaded full, I'd guess 150 to 200 passengers. They were filling every seat quickly and taking off; well, *almost* every seat was filled.

As I got on the plane I went right to the back because again, being that size, I hated being up front where everybody could see me struggling to get into my seat. I went right to the back corner. I sat down, but they couldn't seat anyone next to me, because, once again I was too big. I was taking up too much room. I was spilling over into the next seat. I had the armrest beside me lifted and was taking up two seats. There was another gentlemen in my row of three seats closest to the aisle. I was beside the window. The middle seat was vacant but I was crowding that area.

I LOOKED around the plane and it was completely packed, and as far as I could see, there was only that one empty seat in the entire plane - the one beside me. There was that unforgettable, unmissable half-space beside me.

The whole plane ride, all the way to Edmonton I kept seeing that little space there and I kept thinking about that space which could have held another person if I weren't so huge; about how lonely and miserable I was; how out of bounds my life had become. This thought finally slammed into the centre of my entire being, into every fibre of my conscience: *"Enough is enough!"*

I WAS LOOKING out the window, seeing huge plumes of smoke from the fires filling the northern half of the provinces' skies. I was thinking about the events of the last couple of weeks. I was thinking about how I was taking up two seats. My mind filled with everything negative about my excessive weight in those moments. My mind raced through all of the "What ifs?" I realized that I had gotten out safely and everyone else probably would too, but what if they didn't? Things were going through my mind about how my size was restricting me, how it was hurting my quality of life. I was thinking about everything having to do with my problem with obesity. It was like it was all staring me right in the face and I couldn't ignore it any longer. I couldn't put it off another minute. I could no longer lie to myself. I was done with it. I was convinced that I had enough of it all. Finally.

Questions bounced around my thoughts about what I would do next. What if Fort McMurray burned to the ground and I had nowhere to go? What if I had to get another job? Who would hire me? I reflected on how the camps were not designed for my size. What if I did have to go to work, but we weren't allowed back in Fort McMurray for months? What if I had to live in camp and sleep in that little bed? How would I use the tiny shower? How could I manage being this huge size?

That's when it all clicked. Something changed right in that moment. I haven't been the same ever since because these two words kept rattling around my brain:

"That's. Enough!"

I could hear the words inside my head, over and over again in different forms. "That's enough. This is enough. You either change or your life is done."

It was around supper time when we landed in Edmonton. I got my car from the airport parking and everything already seemed different. I knew things were different and would continue to be different from that point on. After my mind "clicked" on that flight back to Edmonton, after that moment, everything *WAS* different. I remember I went for supper. I can't remember where for sure, but I can remember right then and there I ate healthily. I didn't wait until the next day. I *didn't* have one final meal with extra meat and extra cheese and bacon, extra fries, a side of gravy, two desserts, an extra roll, a Pepsi with unlimited refills; none of that. There was no going for a drive and stopping by a donut shop for a three thousand calorie snack; no treat of chocolate bars or ice cream.

I'm not exactly sure but I think I had a chicken dinner. With the stress of the evacuation, many of the small details like this are blurry. It might have been Swiss Chalet. I either took off the chicken skin or I ordered something without skin, but I remember that there were vegetables. I didn't have bread or potatoes. I remember I didn't touch any junk food; no pop. I think I had water, but from that point on, that was the end of it. No more unhealthy eating; I was done with that.

THAT WAS IT. No more delays. No more excuses. No white sugar. No white flour. No deep-fried food. No junk food. Nothing. Just eating natural. Only eating clean; meat and vegetables. There was no large portion or second helping for me. I had a regular meal. That was it. I said to myself, "I can't keep living life like that."

I'm not sure if it was that evening or the very next day, but I started walking. No putting it off. I didn't buy special shoes or clothes, I just simply started walking every day. That's how it started. I would walk, not run, not jog, not even walk briskly. I just walked. Everyday I would try to push myself a little further even though it was difficult.

I actually stayed in St. Albert that night, a suburb of Northwest Edmonton. After a good sleep, the next day I went to Red Deer. When I got to Red Deer I drove out to Sylvan Lake. That's where I made my short walks a new, consistent part of my life, starting with a painful five minute walk.

That was it. My life was changing, right then, not the next day, or the next week, but right then and there. There was no waiting until the evacuation was over. This was ON!!

During that second evacuation, I stayed in Red Deer for almost three weeks until we were finally allowed back into Fort McMurray in June. It took quite some time to restore electricity and various essential services to make Fort McMurray habitable again, before the evacuation order was lifted.

The people of Alberta, individuals, organizations, businesses and government agencies, were absolutely incredible during the evacuation. Entire cities reached out to us. I consider Edmonton to be a true city of champions with how they reached out and opened their arms. Every city and town across the province was hospitable and kind wherever Fort McMurray people found a roof over their heads at that time.

The Holiday Inn on 170th Street on the West Side in Edmonton and the Marriott Suites in Red Deer both took great care of me. They were all wonderful people. They offered great rates ("Compassion Rates" all the hotels called it) and excellent service.

The Red Cross was even more amazing than I ever would have expected. They gave out any kind of supplies evacuees might have needed. They also gave us gift certificates and emailed money transfers. It was truly unbelievable. Suncor kept our pay cheques coming. I think many of the gas and oil companies did, which shows their wonderful generosity when you think of it. They had to shut down production with no income generated from those projects, but they made taking care of their workers a priority. Wow! I'm amazed by that and I consider myself fortunate and blessed.

Really, the whole country was wonderful. They donated to Fort McMurray millions of dollars through the Red Cross to help us. People could donate at almost any bank or credit union in Canada, and through that The Red Cross distributed that money to us, wherever it was needed. Even the Alberta government helped out the evacuated residents. They gave each resident, a little over $1000. They matched donations to the Red Cross. It was phenomenal.

In Edmonton, I know all I had to do was just show up at some location near the University with a piece of Fort McMurray ID and was instantly given money. Everybody was wonderfully kind and supportive. I'll never forget it.

I didn't take advantage of all the things offered, but if we showed a Fort McMurray ID, many restaurants offered a free meal. Some gave us a free sandwich and drink, others gave us a free burger and fries; NOT free with the purchase of anything, just free! Telus and Shaw communications opened up free wi-fi, had free charging stations, gave away over 1000 mobile phones and offered free pay phones. There were free services to people with medical needs, free products for celiac people, various drugs stores offered help with prescription refills and helped secure items for special needs. At the airport in Edmonton, Tim Hortons was on site giving out free coffee and Timbits to evacuees as they landed. That might not sound like a big thing, but those little familiarities in a time of crisis are unspeakably comforting to people. (Another reason to love Tim Hortons!)

There were free services for pet owners, free storage space for evacuees, free tire repairs, free attractions for families, free clothes, free groceries — the support was truly overwhelming. It almost makes me cry just thinking about how kind people were to the evacuees. Crisis truly does bring out the worst, but also the very BEST in people at times like this. God bless everyone who helped no matter how great or small their contribution. It doesn't go unnoticed or unappreciated. It still touches my heart to this day.

I wanted to be in Red Deer just to be near Emma. I got several offers to stay with Emma's family. They've always been great to me. Even her mother offered me a place to come stay with her. I decided it was best to stay on my own.

My insurance was paying for the hotel and the hotels, as I said, were all offering discounts for displaced Fort McMurray residents. I had a king suite at the Marriott those weeks. It was sixty or seventy bucks a night; certainly a ridiculous bargain. They offered free laundry service, a hot breakfast in the morning and my home insurance coverage from AMA paid for it all.

As I said, I like my space. It's funny because people, old friends, new friends and people I meet, they often say I'm the most stubborn person they've ever met. I think a lot of that comes from being big, being on my own and becoming ruggedly independent. To be that size and to go through my day-to-day life, I had to be stubborn. I had to be independent. I had to say to myself, "I'm here right now, but my car is over there. I'm out of breath but I've got to get there." I had to be stubborn and independent to get around, to function and to make it through life everyday.

Being independent and private helped me protect many of the embarrassing parts of obesity. That's part of the reason why I preferred not to stay in any home, no matter how many times people offered. I was pleased to be alone in a hotel. I had privacy to begin my earliest days of change.

3

From Newfoundland to Fort McMurray

I grew up on the Northern Peninsula of the Province of Newfoundland. My home province is the most easterly region in Canada and North America. I come from a beautiful little town called St. Lunaire-Griquet. It is a little port town right on the Atlantic coast that's home to about six hundred people. It's about a twenty-minute drive from St. Anthony, which is the largest community up there on the Northern Peninsula. St. Anthony, the nearby metropolis, has about 2,000 people. It has a Tim Hortons coffee shop, which is about all I need. Most of the St. Lunaire-Griquet population are older retirees. It was formerly a town of close to 1,200 people back in the early '90s, but when they shut the cod fishery down, a lot of younger people, including myself, moved away.

My Beautiful Village

The home in which I grew up was right on the ocean. When I would wake up in the morning as a boy I could smell the salt water. There were often whales coming into the harbour and in the summertime icebergs would come floating on through our area. Sometimes, lying in bed I'd suddenly hear a great big, explosive bang. It was so loud you might have thought it was a gun going off in the next room or right outside, but it was only the familiar sound of a piece of iceberg breaking off. I'm sure people would pay millions to have a house there in such an idyllic setting and I'm fortunate to say that's where I grew up. Nowadays cruise ships are always coming into that area - it truly is beautiful.

My parents never had much money as I was growing up. We were a family of fishermen. We had our own garden and grew our own fresh vegetables. We had a cow and some sheep, but we fished for a living. It was good, honest work. There was always a lot of work for a fishing family. It was a good life.

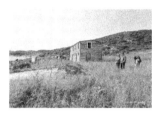

My home town.

We ate like kings. My mom was one of the best cooks I've ever known. Everything we had was homemade; homemade pies, homemade cookies, homemade bread - that homemade bread, oh my goodness! To have a slice of that with some freshly baked beans; that was delicious. All of this was before the days of automatic bread makers. Mom *never* had store-bought cookie dough in our house. Everything was made from scratch.

Our little port town was a five minute drive from where the Vikings first landed in North America, hundreds of years before Christopher Columbus ever saw our continent. They were the first European settlers in North America. I tell people, before you had New York City, before you had Los Angeles, before you had Toronto, you had L'Anse aux Meadows. It's a United Nations Heritage Site. There is a big museum there nowadays drawing tourists from all around the world.

It's a very busy place in the summertime, but absolutely

beautiful. In the wintertime, there is a lot of snow and cold weather. Being right on the ocean you get those strong, harsh winds. It's a hard place to live in the wintertime, but summertime is beautiful. Up the coast, a few hours away we have the Gros Morne Mountains on the one side of the peninsula and the ocean on the other side. The area is filled with fiords (fjords), like something you would see in Scandinavia. It's absolutely gorgeous.

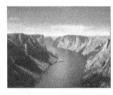
Gros Morne National Park, Newfoundland.

In the Northern Peninsula we would actually have polar bears come from the mainland in the wintertime across the straight from Labrador. They manage to come across on the ice or even swim across; they're actually very strong swimmers. There's one spot where it's only about 20 km from the mainland to the island, not too far for a polar bear to cross.

Fishin' and Boatin'

While I was still in school I fished with my father. I used to love going out fishing with him. There were five of us in his crew. We'd go out to the ocean in my Dad's 30 foot boat. The Newfoundland term for this boat was a "trap skiff". That's what we would use to go out on the cod trap. It was an open boat with an old diesel engine in it. In our boat, everybody had their own spot where they would sit. My dad would always go up in the forward part of the boat. My brother would kind of sit in the middle, another guy would sit in his special spot, it was almost a superstitious thing of habit, everybody sitting where they did and it wouldn't be messed with. I would often get in the back of the boat with one crew member - his name was Roy Bussey - he was a neighbour, a cousin and a close friend. I still go visit him when I'm home. He's older, really old now, but I would sit in the back of the boat with him.

The boat was steered with what was called a *tiller*. The tiller was on the back of the boat and was just a big piece of L-shaped wood, but not even as fancy as a rudder. The crew had a stick that would control the tiller. Dad would take the boat from the wharf and he would go out past a couple rocky areas. Then he would look at me and tap the stick, meaning it was time for me to take over the tiller. He would sit down on the back of the boat and have a smoke. I would stand up, happy as could be. I would get to steer the boat right out to the cod trap.

I loved it. I absolutely loved it. I was just a kid, but I was happy as a clam and proud as could be, like an experienced old fisherman, chin up, standing at the tiller with my nose to the wind. I had to stand up to see over the front of the boat, but when I did I was standing right up behind the exhaust, where the diesel fumes were coming out of the engine. My nose was not really to the wind, it was toward the diesel.

To this day, when I go by a diesel truck, or I'm working and I smell diesel, it brings me right back to those proud moments, holding the tiller. Every time we would go out on the cod trap, I would get to steer. Looking back on it, I think Dad just let me pilot the trap skiff because he wanted to sit down to have a smoke and get away from the diesel fumes, and he probably thought, "Ah, I'll let the kid do it."

I was gone all week long in the summer, up early every morning. There was no showering every day at 5:00 a.m. or any fancy routine. I was only eight or ten years old when I started going out with the fishing crew. At the end of the week, I would have a bath and I would take a face cloth and rub it around my neck. It was as black as black could be, covered in diesel soot. I loved it. To this day, that's a very fond memory, working on the boat, holding the tiller and going out with my father.

I REMEMBER one Saturday night my dad still talks about. Down by the wharfs, everything was pretty much shut down. People were out and about, visiting with each other and enjoying the night. It was a quiet, lovely evening by the ocean. The water was nice and calm. In Newfoundland, they would say "cam, nice and cam." We used to leave a couple of salmon nets out. Dad and I figured, "Let's go check the nets." Salmon at the time was a very valuable catch, still is. If you caught a forty pound Atlantic salmon to sell at five or six bucks a pound…wow! Landing one of those was a nice little payday bonus for the week. That was a lot of money. If you managed to get two or three in the net, it was like Christmas! This salmon net floated on the top of the water. We'd see it floating and go lift it out of the water to see if we had caught anything.

Dad and I, or "me and Dad", as we'd say down home, took a smaller boat and we went out to check the salmon net that Saturday night. He let me steer the boat. It was just me and him. I loved being out with Dad on the water, especially when he let me be the captain. We pulled up to the net. We grabbed it and we pulled the boat along side of it and we looked down to search for our possible prize. If we saw silver in the water, it would mean we got a salmon. On this particular Saturday night, I saw a silver flash. Dad said, "Pull up the net! Pull it up!"

I pulled up the net and sure enough, there was this huge salmon. It had to be close to 40 pounds; a big, beautiful Atlantic salmon. I was right happy! Right away I was figuring, I was calculating, "Holy crap, that's a forty-pounder, five bucks a pound Dad! That's a lot of money."

I could see Dad was right pleased too with a big smile. I proceeded to get the salmon out of the net. As soon as I took the salmon out of the net, it wiggled. Splash! He was gone in a flash, just like that! Two hundred bucks down the drain, or into the ocean at least.

I felt horrible.

I thought Dad was going to be really upset with me. Maybe he saw the look of terror, me holding my breath or the sick look on my face. I don't know. When I looked over at my dad, he just started laughing. As quickly as I felt horrible, I was relieved all at once with his joy and his laughter.

He patted me on the back and I think he said something like, "Ah, it's all right Tony. I've done that a million times." With a smile he said, "We won't say nothin'. Let's just go on in, buddy. We'll go in and enjoy our Saturday night." Dad didn't care. He still talks about that to this day. It's one of my fondest memories of me and my dad.

I HAVE one brother and my mom and dad; just a family of four growing up. My brother still lives back there in Newfoundland. He's three years older than me. He has a couple of boys, so another family of four. All my family is back home in Newfoundland, except my daughter who lives in Red Deer, Alberta. I have no family in Fort McMurray.

It was wonderful growing up in Newfoundland. There's a lot of spectacular scenery right by the ocean; a lot of moose, bears, polar bears, deer, caribou, and smaller game as well. There are many varieties of wildlife around all the time. There is a lot of tourism and even more is forecast with a new highway being built on the mainland through Labrador which will increase accessibility to the Great Northern Peninsula of Newfoundland. With ecotourism a current trend, the beautiful water is an attractive prospect. Amazing as the scenery is itself, seeing the whales amidst it all is breathtaking.

I remember several times being on the water, rowing along

in my little row boat and seeing whales. I remember one day in particular rowing along, hearing the swish, swish sound beside me. I looked over and saw a big ol' freaking humpback whale, maybe 30 feet away. He was just doing his thing, swimming along, peacefully. He floated up to the surface to blow. Dad would always tell me, "Ah, don't worry about those Tony. They're more afraid of you than you are of them."

"Yeah, okay dad, sure." I didn't know it then, but I believe it now. The whales were huge and seemed very scary to me as a young lad.

Most boys would spend a lot of time on their bikes, but I was known around town as the boy always out in the row boat fishing, or just exploring. I was *always* exploring. I loved it!

There's nothing like those memories of being a little boy, especially not knowing how to swim! It was exhilarating to be out of the harbour on the open sea with a mammal the size of a school bus floating by my wee little row boat and checking me out! I'm not so sure those things were *ever* afraid of me. I was only terrified of them!

I used to worry my mom quite a bit, because I'd be off in the row boat, with no cell phones back then, gone exploring all day and she'd have no idea where I was. She'd always say, "Don't go out on the ocean", but I'd go out there anyways. I can't even swim an inch. I'd be out in that little boat. I wouldn't even have a life jacket with me. Mom would yell after me heading out the door, "Take your life jacket", but I'd never take it.

My main childhood memory is that rowboat. I still think about that rowboat. Few things in life make me smile like that rowboat did, or still does for that matter. My dad built me that rowboat when I was a young kid, I think eight or nine years old. I loved it. I think that boat gave me the desire I have in me now to travel, to explore and discover new things. I think it all came from that little boat. I'd get in that little rowboat, and I would row everywhere, anywhere into the great big world. I'd explore all around the big harbour that was in front of my house. Sometimes I even ventured out into the open ocean, beyond the safety of the harbour, without my mother knowing. Out there I would row around all the little coves, the little inlets, just exploring. At that young age, I'd take off by myself, unsupervised. I didn't mind traveling by myself, onto a little beach, I'd light a fire, I'd tour around, tie up my boat somewhere, walk around a bit. They were awe-inspiring adventures for a young boy. It was very peaceful.

As I said, I couldn't swim, foolishly I'd be out in that little boat all day long rarely taking a life jacket along. I remember a couple times, my dad would have to come down to the water to get me out of my rowboat at midnight, down by the wharf. He would come and get me and he'd say, "Come on up! You can go back in your boat tomorrow." Then he'd tie up my boat and we'd head home. To this day, back in my little town, everybody still talks about me and the little rowboat - that kid in his boat. Someday I'm going to have a rowboat again.

My dad has kept my little boat back home. I would like to restore it, or fibreglass it over, to keep it. That was my biggest, my fondest memory of childhood, being in that boat every day. It kept me active and I got plenty of good exercise and fresh air. Spring, summer or fall, if the weather was calm enough, I'd be off in my rowboat, checking my nets, pretending I was a full-on fisherman. I didn't stay in the house much. I was always gone in my boat, gone somewhere on an adventure, fishing, rowing or exploring.

Those are my fondest memories, the rowboat, the water, fishing with my dad. That pretty much explains my long-standing life goal, to retire and live somewhere next to the water; whether that's a big lake, or an ocean, it doesn't matter. That's where I want to wake up in the morning and go out on the porch, the deck, or as we call it in Newfoundland, the "bridge." I'd love to be able to go out on my bridge and sit there, to overlook the water and enjoy my coffee, then maybe jump in my boat, and go exploring for the day; that'd be heaven to me.

MY DAD WAS a cod fisherman pretty much his whole life, since he was a little boy. He's 81 years old right now. He's been retired for many years. My mom worked in a fish plant doing all kinds of different jobs. She also worked for Statistics Canada for a little while. Basically, like many second income earners back home, she'd work at whatever jobs would come up. There aren't many big careers in the little outport towns in Newfoundland. Folks would take whatever job they could pick up at the time. She was a typical Newfoundland housewife and mother. She raised me and my brother, did all of the housework and cooking and worked a bit on the side when she could. My mom is probably the strongest person I know. She's been through a lot in her life, but she never let difficulties keep her down. She would just faithfully get up in the morning and do her thing every day, always carrying that *strong, silent-type* strength. Even today she never complains, never says anything negative, she just gets up every day and gets it done. She's incredibly strong. I don't think you see that in a lot of people anymore. She's very resilient, very tough.

She'd do anything for her family, absolutely anything. She worries a lot. She worries way too much, about everything. I always tease her about worrying, but I can be that way myself at times, worrying a bit too much about things. Dad's more carefree. He's funny, always telling stories. In fact, Dad gets invited to weddings just to tell stories. He likes being social. My mom and my brother, they keep more to themselves, but me and my dad are more social. We love to be out with people enjoying every minute of it.

Faith Background

Both of my parents are good Christian folks. My mom was always a devout Christian lady. Dad wouldn't always go to church. Dad had a problem with drinking there for a while when I was younger, but he gave all that up cold turkey about 25 years ago. He totally stopped drinking and smoking. He started going to church at that time and he hasn't touched alcohol or cigarettes in years.

My dad had two brothers that were both killed tragically many years ago when he was young. I think those events had a very negative effect on him. My one uncle, dad's brother, lived out in Thompson, Manitoba and he drowned. He was only 25 when he drowned. My dad had another brother who was also 25 when he got killed. He worked for Ontario Hydro, from what I remember of the story. He got hit in the back of the head with a boom, from what dad told me, and he was killed.

My poor grandmother found out about one of these tragic deaths over the radio. She was at home doing her dishes in the kitchen and it was announced over the radio that her son had been killed. Back then, I guess it took so long for the information to get back to the family, they didn't yet have that "names are withheld until next of kin are notified" announcement. Dad said she collapsed on the floor with grief. Dad still talks about his brothers to this day. I don't think he's ever gotten over all of the pain and grief associated with the death of his brothers. As hard as those losses were for him Dad eventually moved on from drinking and I'm proud of him for it.

Dad had several sisters as well. One of them, my aunt Velma, is like a second mom to me. She stayed home in Newfoundland along with her husband and they ran the local grocery store in my home town. It's a typical rural village, port-town grocery store where you can buy everything from hardware to lumber, booze, fishing gear, bait and tackle and, oh yes, groceries.

I love going there. Every time I go home, I always go up to the old store. I'll head up three or four times each visit because it's not only a grocery store, it's the local gathering place. Many of the customers hang out and you get to see people from all around the area. All of my cousins run the place now. It's called the "Burden's General Store." They're wonderful people. Whenever I visit the store they give me hugs and smiles and sit down with me to catch up. It's wonderful to be back home.

I went to a Pentecostal church growing up. In Newfoundland, they have the smallest towns where they have huge Pentecostal churches. The Pentecostal church in my hometown probably owns most of the town. The church building holds 400-500 people; a massive seating capacity that can almost hold the entire population. It's a huge, modern church built back in about 1990; a beautiful facility. I grew up in the Pentecostal church where I went to church and Sunday school and the youth group in my teen years.

In Newfoundland the big church service is not on Sunday morning like the rest of Christian churches in the world. It's the Sunday *evening* service that everybody attends. The morning service is the smaller and usually more traditional service. Everybody wants to get home for the big Sunday dinner. In Newfoundland, the big Sunday meal is not supper, it's dinner. Families have the big meal at 12 o'clock, a huge fancy spread. Sunday supper is usually a small little meal, just a snack.

Sunday night church, however, was larger than life. I remember walking into church and the place would be packed. Coming into the building you'd notice everybody dressed up in their finest clothes, suits and ties or their nicest dresses, the whole "Sunday best" thing. I remember walking into the sanctuary and even before I got inside, I would hear the people gathered up at the front, the elders of the church, praying. They would be "calling down heaven" actually, not just silent prayers, but loud and "fervent" prayers, passionate and filled with emotion. The prayer time before church wouldn't be in a private room, it'd be right there in the main gathering room of the church. The whole community would be there. The place was electric. It was a nice feeling.

As the service started the lively music would kick in. I think I got my love of music from these times. There would be somebody on piano, on the guitar, on the drums and there was always somebody playing accordion. The place would really be animated with lively music, gospel songs. You wouldn't see it as much now, but back then, somebody would always have the accordion going. Then somebody else would get up and lead the singing and the whole place would come to life. Sunday night there would be a "testimony time" as part of the evening service; it was an absolute necessity to have those testimonies in a Sunday night Pentecostal Newfie service.

I took in one of these Sunday evening services when I was back home this past summer, with my mom. Sure enough, they still have the testimony service. In a testimony service, folks will just stand to their feet and talk about how thankful they are for God's help, or how He's answered prayer, or how their lives have been transformed with God's help. For some of these dear souls, it's been the exact same testimony they share once a month or every few months, or goodness, sometimes every week for years on end.

THERE WAS one repeated story I remember well, some poor

man, he had something go wrong with his health, but God had healed him. Every Sunday, he would get up to remind us. It was his white blood cell count, or something along those lines. He would get up every Sunday and word for word it would be the same exact testimony. I remember that as a kid. He passed away years ago now. He used to say something like "I just gotta stand and give da' Lord glory, give him tanks and praise." ("Tanks" is Newfie for "thanks"). He'd go up and down with his voice. He had the same tone and emphasis every time he told the old story. Then he would clap. Then he would shout a few times, then clap again. Then he'd stamp his foot. Then he'd sit down. Then most everybody else in church would chime in like it was the first time they were hearing his recollections saying, "Amen brother, amen." Those were special memories. It's really something to see. It's beautiful how grateful and appreciative these folks are for every little blessing in the middle of their difficulties and problems.

IT BRINGS BACK a lot of memories. That's where I was as a kid, staying out of trouble, sitting in church. A lot of times, I'd be sitting in a church service, bored, just marking up a hymn book, drawing pictures of boats.

I enjoyed the serenity of Sundays. Back then, Sunday was a day of rest. I couldn't go in the boat on a Sunday. I wasn't allowed. I couldn't work on Sunday, no one could; even to this day, my father doesn't even like *shaving* on a Sunday.

My father told stories of the fishery from when he was a child. The fishery was a lot busier then. There used to be more fish prior to the moratorium, decades before the fishery closed down. Saturday evening, they would be working at the fishery until late but they had to time it just right so they wouldn't be working past midnight. If they couldn't have all the work done by then, the remaining fish were thrown overboard because no one wanted to be caught working past 12:00 a.m.. Technically it was Sunday, the "Lord's Day", a day of rest. No one could be unloading, packing, moving or guttin' fish on the Lord's day!

Dad said it seldom got that close to midnight, but sometimes it did. If they had to, they would shut it all down right before midnight.

Sunday, no one would fish. As they'd say on the Rock, "no one did nut'in'!" We tied up our boats Saturday night. We would get cleaned up and be done with any kind of work until Monday morning. It had been tradition for generations.

In the old days they would come up to the house Saturday night and open the doors with Newfie hospitality. It would often turn into a house party with all the lights on, music playing and food flowing through the house, everywhere. My grandmother would be carrying on with a fiddle playing and they'd all be singing hymns, or singing the old Newfie songs. People would be over to the house eating, laughing and having fun, but they would *never* work after midnight.

Sunday was special. We'd always enjoy a home cooked meal. Sunday afternoon was nap time. I loved Sunday evening. Sunday was church. Sundays, as I said, we would have our big cooked dinner near noon, then later we'd all be at church Sunday night, then Monday we would get back in the boat again. That was life!

I'd be looking down toward the water, staring at my boat all day Sunday, longing for it. I couldn't wait to get back out there, especially if the water was calm, a perfect rowing day, but no! I could *never* go out in the boat, not on Sunday.

I didn't fight it. It was what it was. I accepted it. It was the tradition in every family. It was everywhere in Newfoundland. In a way I long for those days again, because now Monday, Sunday, Friday it's all the same. Working shift work, the busy society we work and live in, there's no special "day of rest" any more, no family-focused, quiet-time these days.

I remember we studied the theological concept of a "day or rest" or "sabbath" one time in college. In the Bible God commanded his people to have a day of rest. Sabbath was all about rest, not religious ceremony. It was more so that God knew that we as people needed one day off a week. It seemed to me to be mostly a caring, healthy piece of advice really, more than a heavy commandment, "Here, take a day off, you need this!"

To this day, Sundays feel different to me, whether I work or not, there's a different feeling about Sunday. Back in those days of boyhood it was simpler and quieter. It was peaceful. I don't know if it was Sunday that was so special or perhaps it was the combination of quiet Sundays with the little town that I was in, northern Newfoundland, with all the family right there, the closeness of it. It was beautiful.

I miss the simplicity. I think about those quieter, family-focused days. It makes me smile. It was nice.

For me, Church felt like a safe place. Even now, if I go into the church there is something warm and comforting about the familiarity and the tradition of it. There were people that seemed to be a part of the furniture there, especially fisherman that we would see working all week long and then in church every Sunday. They would be praying and worshipping, good God-fearing men and women. It felt very much like family. These were people that I knew and respected my entire life. I went to school with their kids or grandkids all through the week. Those students were my best friends and peers.

All the older people back then, whether we were related to them or not, they were family. We would call them "aunt" and "uncle" out of respect. "There's uncle George", or "there's aunt Marge." Even though we likely were not related to them at all, we addressed them with that kind of respect. Those people would look out for each other. They would have our backs no matter what might come our way. Even now, when I go back to Newfoundland and visit that church building that has been there almost 30 years, I feel right at home. I step into that building and I feel like I go straight back to those moments when I was a child, almost like time travel.

It feels safe, like sanctuary.

If I see those seniors now, I still call them "uncle" and "aunt." When I approach them, I give them a big hug and it's all smiles. It's fine even though sometimes they don't recognize me until I tip them off and they say, "Oh Tony! How's Tony?" I really value and respect those dear seniors. They all were and still are the pillars of that community, pillars of our society.

I HAD THIS ONE SPECIAL "UNCLE," Uncle Garlan. He was everybody's uncle. When I was a kid, he was in his nineties. He was a special and wonderful man. He was a hundred-and-five-years-old when he finally died in his sleep quite a few years ago. He had two wives who predeceased him. He wanted to fight in World War One, enlisting near the end of the war. By the time he made it clear across the province to St. John's to get on the ship to go overseas, the war was over. It wasn't an easy trip to go from where I lived in the Northern Peninsula, all the way down there to St. John's. It still is a long trip!

Uncle Garlan and I would sit together outside and watch the world go by. I still laugh when I think how if somebody walked by, he'd tap me on the knee and say things like, "Look at this one, Tony. He's stunned!" Then he'd shout at the passerby, "Stunned!" Uncle Garlan would just randomly poke fun at people and he could get away with it at his age.

We would spend a lot of time together, a whole lot of unhurried time together. He'd frequently come over to the house and pick me up. Sometimes he'd get both my brother and me, and we'd go do things together. We would help him cut up some wood, or help him with the fishery. He was very active, even at that age. He had all kinds of stories to tell. He wore suspenders, bullet-style dress pants and usually wore a smile as well.

We would go off on an adventure on the ocean, Garlan and me. He had a little sail boat. We had an old sail which we had made ourselves for that old boat. We'd make our way across the harbour, to go what they called "trouting." We would take our *bamboos* and go catch some trout. I used to love going with Uncle Garlan for cook ups after the trouting. We'd sail clear across the harbour for a cook up. He'd be smoking one of those old style pipes all the while. The memories of the smell of that pipe are warm and inviting.

One time we had a little cook up for the two of us that I remember clearly. On this particular cook up, he brought some caplin to eat. He had the fire lit, and he put the caplin on a stick, put it over the fire and cooked up our lunch; fish roasted on a stick, like something you'd see in a movie or read about in some old novel. I was devouring them. I loved those caplin, a delicious little fish. I was eating away, one mouthful after another. I had plenty of homemade bread and jam to compliment the caplin.

My uncle Garlan was sitting there, smoking his pipe, but he wasn't saying anything. He kept looking over at me and just continued smiling, a half-smile almost. I thought he was eating, and I kept eating away. The poor man sat there for quite some time, patiently waiting for this hungry kid to finish eating. When I did finally eat my fill, we went trouting after the cook up, fishing all afternoon. After a full afternoon, we came all the way across the harbour, got back ashore and headed back home. He came inside the house when we arrived back home. Once inside, the first thing he did was ask my mom to make him a lunch, because he was "starving." Apparently, I ate all of the food, but he didn't say a word. He kept looking over at me and smiling during the cook up. I had no idea that I had eaten all of the provisions that afternoon.

He died a few years ago. I never made it to his funeral. He gave me something memorable years ago, a little letter I have at home; a note he wrote to me that I have held on to as a keepsake. It has great sentimental value to me. Those are very fond memories, times with Garlan.

Working at Home

With the fishery, it was very busy. There were always people around and there were lots of chores for us to do. If we boys weren't involved in the fishery, we were often cutting grass for the sheep. We kept a few sheep. Mom would actually take the wool off of them and ship it away to have it processed. We would use the sheep for food too. We would kill a couple every year, and that was part of how we ate. We also had to tend to the gardens all summer long. It was a lot of work to keep a family fed and sheltered on a budget.

We would cut the tall grass for the sheep and then had to spread the grass out to dry in the sun, then turn it over again later in the day. We had an old scythe and cut all the grass by hand, using a fork to flip it, dry it out and turn it into straw instead of seeing it turn moldy.

Flipping the grass throughout the day kept us busy. At the end of the day we'd lay out big nets on the ground. Using a prong we spread all the drying grass into nets and then tied the nets across themselves corner to corner, bundling them up. It was fun to throw those huge bundles of grass on my back or my brothers' and carry it to the stable overnight. The next day, we would take all the grass out, spread it back out on the field and let it dry again. That one chore alone was almost enough to keep us occupied all summer long.

Along with the grass it was our job to take our sheep over to the other side of the harbour on some pasture land to eat the grass there. The sheep were allowed to roam around all summer grazing. In the fall my brother and I would go get them, chase them around, catch them and bring them back home where they would be fed plenty of carefully dried out grass, hay, for them to enjoy all winter.

WE WERE BROUGHT up to respect nature, the land and the sea. We never killed anything for fun. If we'd go hunting, we wouldn't go hunting for fun. We would hunt for food and that's it. Dad had a high level of respect for the animals. He hated seeing anything hurt or wasted; he couldn't stand that. We'd set snares for rabbits to catch and eat them. All of our meat was fresh. There was rarely anything purchased from the store. I don't ever remember one time when we bought meat from the store. We always had plenty of fresh meat. Of course the fish was always fresh and we even enjoyed lobster every once in a while.

I'LL PROBABLY GET ARRESTED for saying this, but as a boy I used to leave nets out and I'd often catch a few flat fish, tiny little fish and they are literally just flat. They're the funniest looking things with two eyes on the same side. They're actually an Atlantic halibut, a "right-eyed flounder". We'd bring them down to the wharf and sell them. Every once in a while I would accidentally catch a lobster in my net and I wouldn't be disappointed to find one there. I would bring the lobster out and hide it right away. People weren't allowed to catch lobster without a licence. If I did net one I'd pull it out and I'd hide it away in my jacket to smuggle home. It's a wonder I never got pinched by those nasty claws hiding them in my coat.

Looking out through the kitchen window, Mom would see me coming home. I'd be pointing at my coat trying frantically and quietly to tell her about my catch. From a distance in my excitement, I'd be whisper-shouting, "Lobster! Lobster!" I was more so mouthing those words to be more accurate.

She'd give me the angry index-finger-to-her-lips shush signal through the window for fear of somebody finding out or reporting me. In the meantime she'd put a big pot of water on to boil before I was even in the door. We would have a sweet little feed of lobster for supper on those nights. My uncle was a fisheries officer who lived just a couple doors down from us. We always had to keep my accidental little lobster harvests quiet. If I get arrested because of this story, well, it was a good run!

I wonder if there's a statute of limitations on lobstering as a minor? I can see the headlines now, "Former huge man gets arrested after police discover written lobster confession. RCMP and ministry of fisheries officials show up to drag away man who lost 337 pounds immediately after TV interview for eating contraband lobster when he was eight years old."

I was a minor, so maybe I'll be okay. Mom and Dad will probably get arrested for harbouring a minor in the black-market lobster smuggling industry. I can just imagine my poor Mom, getting arrested for boiling water with the crown attorney saying she's an accessory to lobster, feeding her kids and cooking crustacean for them.

We had some really good stories and memories growing up in Newfoundland. Those times are some of the fondest and happiest times of my entire life.

In the wintertime, we cut wood for heat. A lot of people still burn wood back home. It would be ridiculously expensive to heat a home without any firewood in those bitter, cold winters. Every late fall or into the wintertime we would cut all our wood for the year. There'd be a lot of outdoor time to get ready for the cold season. Our home would need about twenty truckloads of wood.

Even to this day, a lot of people down east burn wood to heat their homes. My parents have found a company that will bring in transport trucks full of wood. My mom will pay about $600 for a truck to deliver a full load of wood, already cut. They'll just drop off the wood right there in our yard. Usually my brother will come over and stow it away for them. Then my folks will have wood all winter.

When we were kids and teenagers, forget about spending $600 on wood, we'd do it all ourselves. Oil was too expensive to heat our home all winter. We'd get the wood ready for winter ourselves and save the money, cutting down trees, chopping and hauling wood out in the bush; those made for a lot of good memories.

Summer was definitely the best, being out in the boat, but wintertime was very nice too. We always found something fun to do. On snowy days or nights we would go to our friends homes to go out on a Ski-Doo. Down home back in the day, regardless of brand, every snowmobile would be called a "Ski-Doo." We'd take off on a Ski-Doo, go out into the woods and maybe get a camp fire going out in the bush.

I haven't been "Ski-dooing" for years now, but I understand that in Newfoundland these days they have groomed trails going everywhere, criss-crossing the province. Any Ski-Doo rider can hop on a groomed, mapped trail and go all the way to St. John's if you want. Nowadays I hear the trails even have restaurants and shops along the way, where you can stop in, gas up, grab bite to eat and warm up before you head out again. As kids in the Northern Peninsula, we were far from that kind of organized and groomed trail-riding. We'd just have a simple fire in the woods that we rode to on an old Ski-Doo and that was considered to be wonderful fun for us.

―

WE DIDN'T HAVE much money. We worked for a lot of what we had. We worked to literally put food on the table, not cash in our pockets, but we worked for actual meat, straw, firewood, wool, rabbit and fish. It was definitely a great life though. The house was always spotless, the food was always delicious. We had everything we ever needed. It's not like city life where people have everything at their fingertips; where we go on vacations and fly around the world to make it through the year. I'll elaborate on this more shortly, but when I went off to college, it was my first time out of the province! Most people I knew never went on a vacation to some distant place. We never went really anywhere like that. Winter was cold and in the summer we fished. That was it!

When I got a bit older, I got involved in the church youth group where we'd go off on a youth retrieve, we'd go away a few hours drive to Hawke's Bay on the other side of the peninsula, or some other outing. I remember, in grade ten or eleven, the youth group went into St. John's; we took the bus to get there. It was a huge deal. That was the first time I'd ever seen a movie in a theatre. The trip to St. John's was an eleven hour bus ride, right from one tip of the province to the other end. That's all I had ever travelled, just clear across the island.

Family was important growing up on "the Rock" one of the most common nicknames for Newfoundland. Dad struggled a lot with drinking earlier on in my childhood. That was always hard to deal with. He's strong. He gave it up cold turkey and as I got older. I understood why he wrestled with it. We were in a fishery town where he was not making much money. After the fishery closed down he still had bills to pay, a family to raise and the stress that brings. Then, on top of that, Dad had the grief of having his two brothers pass away and other losses as well. Dad didn't talk about such things very often, not until I got older did he start to talk about any of that. It wasn't an easy life.

When I said there wasn't much money, I only realized that later in life. I found out those stories after I moved away. When I was a kid I would ask Mom for money to go out to the local arcade to play some video games. A lot of times, Mom would give me the last $10 she had. Growing up, dad would put gas in the truck, but it was never a full tank. It was always up to Mom how much cash she would give him, like $5 or $10 to put some gas in the tank. I thought that was normal. I came to find out later it was because they never had money to put a full tank of gas in the truck. Things were tight.

I don't put any gas in my car unless I'm going to fill it right up. I wouldn't put $20 in or some amount short of a fill-up, especially after the Fort McMurray fires. I make sure I have a full tank any time I'm getting gas. I have learned becoming a man to really appreciate all that I've had, as I have seen what my parents went through, the sacrifices they made. Now I have to manage my own home, my bills and my own problems. I'm grateful I have a lot of good memories. I have learned the value of sacrifice and the price people have to pay to get things done well. Willingness to sacrifice has become an important value to me, especially in a society that quickly uses convenient credit for instant gratification. To value sacrifice is a gift given to me by hard working, honourable people; my parents.

My dad mostly retired after the fisheries closed down. The moratorium on codfish happened back in July of 1992. It put about 30,000 people in the province out of work, mostly people who had fished their entire lives, like my dad. The government helped when they "bought back" a lot of the fishing licenses. A fishing license was and still is very hard to get, but when you had one, you basically had it for life. The government offered a buy-back program where they bought the licenses for a big price. Once that license was sold, that was it! You could never fish again. It was almost like a pension for thousands of "forced retirements".

Fishermen all over Newfoundland used the buy-back program money as their pension. My Dad retired and my Mom kept working at a bed and breakfast for years. She recently retired from that, six or seven years ago. After the fishery shut down, the local economy struggled. A lot of young people left and continued to leave in the coming decades; not just my town, but everywhere in Newfoundland, these outport villages continue shrinking. When I grew up I wanted to be a fisherman, going to the cod fishery and making an honest living. Kids can't have that dream now. The fish are gone.

EVERY TIME I go head back to the island, I'll go down to the ocean and sit by the beach. It's sad. You see all the quiet little fishing stages and wharfs and all kinds of collapse. Nobody is fishing anymore since the cod fish moratorium in the early 90's.

I reflect on all the memories of my childhood and all the people that were a part of the landscape decades ago. A lot of those people have now passed away; it's pretty lonely back there, especially since many of the younger generation have moved away like I did.

Every year for my birthday, my mom would make my favourite food. My favourite cake was a spice cake. She'd make that for me as a birthday tradition. My favourite food was this: she would cut up potatoes very thin. I used to call them "floppy discs." She fried them in pork fat which gave it a nice flavour; very greasy, but very thin and floppy. (I'm not sure if you've picked up on this, but before the last two and a half years of my life, I wasn't really a health nut.) Mom would spend hours preparing. She would spend the entire day cooking. As fast as she was as cooking them, I'd be eating them. They were more like a floppy potato chip than a scalloped potato. They would get mostly crispy, deep-fried and hard on the outside, but the inside would be a bit soft and bendable. I can almost taste it now. She'd make me those all day, then she'd make battered fish, always my favourite, cod fish, the way only Mom makes it. Holy crap, that was good! Then spice cake with ice cream afterward; my annual birthday feast.

When I go home now, one of my favourite meals is still baked cod fish that my mom has made the same way as long as I can remember. Mom would clean a cod fish and stuff it like you would a turkey and then bake it with onions and everything else, all the trimmings. We lived well, we ate well and we enjoyed life growing up back east.

School

Not only did I go to a Pentecostal church, I went to a Pentecostal *school* as well. They had Pentecostal separate schools in Newfoundland at the time, so I attended from Kindergarten to grade 12 right there in my home town. "A. Garrigus Collegiate", it was called.

A lot of it was the same as public school, but we would have a few courses about faith, bible, church history and other Christian courses. Usually, we would have prayer in the morning. We would have an assembly, almost like church, once a week. It was good. A lot of our teachers would also be on the church board and involved at church, especially the principal. It was a small school. I know that schools across Canada can be huge; thousands of students. I was in the same building from kindergarten to grade twelve at the little school where I attended. I can't imagine there were more than 200 students in the whole school, K-12. It was the same class of 15 or 20 of us, the same bunch for 13 full years. It was a great experience.

It was only a four or five minute walk from my house to school, so I'd walk home for dinner and then walk back to school for the afternoon. I liked to go to the convenience store near the school to buy a big bag of gum and give it out at school.

I used to love buying chips and if I bought the good chips, everybody would want some of my chips. I started buying Dill Pickle chips and, honestly, I couldn't stand Dill Pickle chips, but nobody else could either. If I bought those, I would have a full bag of chips to myself.

I think that's where I developed my taste for fast food, sweets and snacks, growing up in Newfoundland. Mom would make all kinds of delicious cookies, treats, pies and desserts. I wouldn't have eaten better even if our family were all millionaires. Every once in a while, we'd go up to the *shop*, which is what we call it at home, we call a store a "shop". We would go to the shop and get a bag of chips and a drink. A *can of drink* we would call it. We wouldn't call it a *pop* or a *soda*, we'd call it a can of drink. We'd go to the shop and grab some chips and a can of drink and walk to school. I could have said that earlier, but I felt I needed to teach you some basic Newfie language skills first.

In the Fall of the year, Dad would actually keep me out of school for the first week to help him with the fishery. There was me and one other guy in school who were exempted from classes for fishery reasons. After that week, I would be in school, but I'd get up in the early in the morning and go to the fishery with Dad before the school day. I'd come back home after a few hours of work. My brother would make me breakfast and then I would go on to school after that. I've been getting up since 5:00 in the morning for many years. I loved the fishing life. I was made to get up and head to that water. I used to hate having to go to school and I hated leaving the water. There has always been something pulling me to the water.

Pentecostal school was good. I managed to make it through school and I *mostly* graduated. At that point I remember my mother talking to me and saying I should wait until I was a little older before going off to college. I was stubborn then. I did not listen to her wisdom. I applied for bible college in Peterborough, Ontario, but I still needed one more credit to get in. I needed to finish my math credits to graduate. I remember that the principal in the school tutored me to get it done and with his help I finished it. Gary Davis was his name. He still lives back there; a wonderful gentleman. He helped me graduate, and then I was accepted into bible college.

I look back at pictures of me in grade twelve and I look pretty normal. I look like an average kid. I have pictures on my phone, photos with my mom and dad. I looked like an average-sized student in the twelfth grade. I didn't leave high school huge, maybe a bit overweight, but not big. I'd say I was an average size.

I had a wonderful childhood; pretty good I'd say. I have plenty of good memories and stories. I realize now that food is a significant part of the culture in Newfoundland, but obviously, not every Newfie is obese. I know for me, many times, all of those delicious foods were often viewed as a reward, because many times that's all there was. There was no movie theatre nearby to go to; no bowling alley; no laser tag; no go-kart track; no theme park; no Disney or wonderland within a quick commute. A good part of the social life down east is just being invited over to someone's house or popping over for tea, cookies and pie.

I'm not making an excuse, but because there was nothing else to do in my little town, I developed a mentality that would come back to haunt me - *food as a reward, as entertainment, as a treat.*

No matter how much or how little we had, every household we went into, there was always food. There was always delicious food. I thought it was normal to have sweets, pies and cakes. It's almost like I grew up thinking, "Whether I do well or do poorly, there's always food." If I was having a bad day, a cookie or a brownie consoled me. If I was having a good day, I'd have a nice bowl of pea soup and crackers, comfort food to enjoy the end of a good day. I'm not saying this to blame anyone or anything, but all my life, food has been one of these two things: a comfort or a celebration.

I never did drugs. I never drank. Seeing what my dad went through with alcohol completely turned me off of that, especially to ever think of getting drunk. I've tried alcohol, but I rarely drink the stuff. I might have it once every few years or so. Once in a blue moon I might have a couple drinks. Generally speaking, I don't drink. I've seen what it's done to my mother. When my Dad was drinking, they would fight quite a bit over it. Mom hated it when Dad would come home drunk. When he drank he'd be angry, or miserable. It's not worth it to me.

My memories of my childhood could not be much better. My parents are wonderful people that I honour and I still have a world of respect for them both. I left them in 1993 to go tackle the world all on my own.

From High School to Fort McMurray

I headed off to Bible College from 1993 to 1996. Since I had gone to a Pentecostal Church my whole life, since I was part of a Pentecostal school system starting in kindergarten and since faith was a positive part of my life, it didn't seem to be a bad idea to head off to Bible College. Our denominational Bible

School was in Peterborough, Ontario, Eastern Pentecostal Bible College or EPBC, or just "Eastern" for short.

I enrolled in the 4 year bachelors of theology degree program, because then perhaps down the road I would have been able to get a job teaching in the Newfoundland Pentecostal school system or goodness knows, I maybe could have even become a minister, anywhere in Canada for that matter. The 4-year Bachelor of Theology (BTh) could open doors for teaching in my home province but potentially it could also open the door to being a pastor anywhere across Canada. The accompanying internship and then credentialing process could make that possible. Why not try it? I even felt some sense of *calling*.

Looking back on it, I sometimes have regrets about going after the BTh degree. Part of the course requirement is to take a full year of one of the Biblical languages, either Hebrew or Greek. Contrary to my instincts and my inner feelings about languages, I decided to take Hebrew. I attempted to take that a few times, and I just could not get it. That frustration eventually led me to leaving college, but let me tell you more about those years.

I was 18 when I left home in 1993. I'd never been off the island of Newfoundland at that point. I had never been anywhere. Here I was, an 18-year-old, leaving a tiny little outport in northern Newfoundland to fly to Toronto, Ontario, a world class city with 6.4 million people in the greater Toronto area (GTA), North America's forth largest city.

At that time, my uncle was living in Scarborough, Ontario, an east end suburb. He picked me up at the airport. I was an isolated Newfie kid landing at the Toronto airport, which was a whole other world to me. It might as well have been landing on a different planet. I remember being mesmerized by all the big tall buildings. I was amazed by it all taking it in like a tourist.

My uncle drove me to Peterborough, 100 km east of Scarborough. He took me to the EPBC campus, a wonderful facility, beautiful grounds, lovely park space, an incredible location. Everyone there at the orientation was a first year. I was there completely by myself, but I felt right at home. Being a first year from Newfoundland at EPBC has a great advantage. There's a large student population from the island. It was a very manageable transition.

I became life-long friends with some of those people I met that first year. I still talk to them to this day. A few of them even moved up to Fort McMurray. I met my friend Chad Perry there, a friend for life. We've known each other for well over 20 years. Other friends, Mark Baker and Dana Head are up there too. Dana actually works at the same company as me, Suncor. I see him there all the time.

Outside of growing up in a Newfoundland fishery, I look back at that time, those first few years of college, as one of the best times of my life. Whenever I'm in Ontario, I try to make a point of renting a vehicle and visiting friends I made in the college years.

I lived in residence for most of my time at college, but there was a time I stayed in a house with a few other guys who had a house rented. Dorm life was perfect; good cafeteria, comfortable rooms. For me it was probably better just being fresh out of Newfoundland, I didn't know anything about living on my own.

That was before the days of cell phones. I couldn't afford to have a landline in my room, although I probably should have, looking back on it. I put so much change in pay phones it would have paid for a phone I'm sure. I'd have to call collect to talk with Mom. Times were tight. I remember I had a student loan, but that only covered the basics. I had cafeteria food, but being in college, I'd always want a pizza with friends, or I'd want to go out for a bag of chips. Often a bunch of friends would want to go to Haaseltons Café downtown Peterborough and have a coffee or something and not having much money I'd hit Mom up for cash.

I'd call Mom from the payphone, a collect call and request a donation. I remember there was a Royal Bank at the Chemong Plaza near the school that would dish out $5 bills from their ATM. Mom would put in $40 or $50 for me. I could walk there while she'd be driving up to the RBC in St. Anthony, which is a 20-minute drive away where she'd deposit some cash into my account. When she would hang up, she would leave the house to drive while I'd walk twenty minutes to the RBC in Peterborough. I would put my bank card in the ATM and it would say, "insufficient funds." I would wait a little longer. We had no cell phones yet, so I'd constantly be looking at my watch, a device strapped to my wrist that would tell me the current time. I'd wait another ten minutes, and I'd put my bank card back in and then I'd hear, "Ching, ching, ching, ching, ching," as the money would be dispensing. What a magical sound. Then I'd head right next door to the convenience store for some snacks or across the road to KFC and have some serious chicken.

I started my journey of weight gain at college. I was a bit bigger than average then, not huge, but I was on the heavy side. I wore an XL in college or even an XXL, but I could still easily find clothes at Zellers or Walmart or any men's shop. I could still buy suits and dress clothes.

I remember one summer in college I lost weight. I lost about 80 - 90 pounds. I didn't keep the weight off. The thing that I did differently then that I'm not doing now, is I went back to a mentality of "treating" myself. I still would have "treats." I finished a paper, I thought I deserved a treat. If I made it through a week of classes, I thought I deserved a bag of chips. If I passed an exam, "Let's go for ice cream!" I have never changed my lifestyle as much as I have in the last two-and-a-half years. I lost the weight quickly in college, but I never changed a thing about my lifestyle. I have learned since then that dieting and lifestyle change are two totally different things.

I didn't know much about diet or healthy eating or lifestyle while I was in college, I just put the weight back on that I had lost that one summer. It certainly didn't take long for me to regain *all* the weight I'd lost over the next couple years. A lifestyle that considers food as a treat, as a comfort or as a central part of socialization is bound to bite you in the butt — or make that butt grow.

After three years of college, I left. I wasn't able to just get a three year diploma because I wasn't in the diploma program. The course structure was too different from the BTh degree, so I left with nothing; no degree and no diploma. That's frustrating and it was all because of one choice I made when I signed up for a degree with a language requirement.

Then I went to work. I worked for Burns Security in Peterborough, at the old Johnson & Johnson factory. It's ironic because a Pentecostal church ended up buying that property and it is now Calvary Church. After that, I worked for a window installation company. I took out another student loan and went back to bible college figuring, "At least I wanna try to finish this."

I only had one year left. I really wanted to finish my bachelors degree. After another full year, I still couldn't get past that Hebrew language course. I never did complete it. Sometimes I look back and I think, "What kind of path would life have taken if I had a degree or a diploma? Would I have gotten a teaching job or a job in a church?" Only God knows.

When I got working steadily it was often convenient to eat out all the time. I slowly started to pack on extra pounds. The diet of convenient fast-food wiped out any gains I had a few summers earlier with weight loss.

After a while I got frustrated with living in Peterborough,

because I wasn't making much money. I was at another window company and I went to ask for a raise. I was only making eight bucks an hour, working two jobs. I was getting tired of it. My supervisor asked me, "How much money do you want to stay at it?"

I told him I would stay for ten dollars an hour. The supervisor went to the owner, then came back relaying the response, "Well, if Tony doesn't like it, then there's a whole stack of resumes there."

I gave them two weeks notice and then I left. I threw everything in my car. I didn't have any money to do it, but I had a friend in Peterborough, Lisa Bapty. Her mother helped me out. That wonderful lady was really involved in the church and she kindly gave me $300, so I could afford to go out west and look for a job.

I had an old, little, yellow Geo Metro, all beat up. I put everything I had in a couple of garbage bags and drove out west. There was talk of decent paying jobs out in the oil sands, so I thought I'd give it a shot. That was 1999.

By the time I got to Fort McMurray, I was about 340, 350 pounds. Fort McMurray was where I really ballooned, I got huge in Fort McMurray over the next 16 years.

Fort McMurray and Emma

Arriving in Fort McMurray I worked another job before I got hired on with Suncor December 10th, 2001. I lucked out to get the job because I had some limited experience driving a big vehicle. The oil sands have plenty of huge vehicles so that looked good on my resumé. I'm very thankful to have settled in Fort McMurray because I have a great job, I have a great life and it opened a door for Emma to come into my life.

Emma means the world to me. She's sort of my "stepdaughter," but I consider her to be my daughter. I first met

Penny, Emma's mom, when I moved to Fort McMurray. Penny lived there with her family. I met her through a mutual friend. Penny is a wonderful lady. She's been through a lot in her life, but came through the difficulties a strong and determined woman. After I had known her for about a year, she broke up with the guy she was dating. After that she found out she was pregnant with Emma, which to me was not an issue. Penny and I started dating while she was pregnant with Emma. I was actually in the room with Penny watching the whole thing unfold when Emma was born; I got to cut Emma's cord!

I was in the delivery room by Penny's invitation with her and her sister. Emma's real dad wasn't in the picture and he hasn't really been in the picture at all through her life. I was pretty close with Penny and her family. I still am really. They're a wonderful family. I can't say enough good stuff about them. They're funny. They're a bunch of characters. They'll give you the shirt off their backs - those kind of people. I could go to Red Deer tomorrow and say, "I need a place to stay," and any one of her sisters would invite me in without hesitation, in a moments' notice.

Most of the family have moved to Red Deer now. I still go down there, about a six hour drive, to visit Emma. It's not awkward visiting Penny, my former girlfriend. Penny got married. Her husband is a terrific guy. When I go to Red Deer to visit Emma, I often go in to their place and I visit with Penny and her husband. We'll sit down and have a coffee or a bite to eat. They're terrific people.

I like Penny's husband. His name is George. I like to tease Penny and tell her, "The only reason I'm coming to visit is because I like George better." They are fun to hang out with and great for Emma.

Emma was born on February the seventh, 2001. I dated her mom for about four years. It was love at first sight with Emma. To me she was a wonderful child. In the end, dating her mom didn't work out — stuff happens right? However, I stayed in Emma's life. I couldn't leave her. Emma had my heart. There was no way I could walk away from her. She has been my daughter ever since she was born.

Staying connected with Emma was difficult at first. Obviously, Penny and I had just broken up. Her mother had moved on, but I would still go over and visit Emma and take her out. We'd go for meals together. We'd go to movies. I'd take her to the park, push her on the swings or go to a mall and maybe buy her a little gift. We stayed close. I tried to see her as much as I could being the significant male role model in her life in Fort McMurray. During my days off from work, I would pick her up for an afternoon, not every day, but at least a couple times each week. Penny still welcomed me as the father figure in Emma's life.

The only problem Penny had was with me giving Emma too much junk food. That was her only issue. Penny would lecture me and say, "Don't give Emma so much junk food." When Emma and I would go out she'd say things like, "Dad, we're going to have junk food, right?"

Wrapped around her finger I would say, "Oh, yeah. For sure." I remember how Emma would laugh about that and still laughs about it to this day because I would tell Emma, "Never lie to your mother…but you don't have to give her any information she doesn't need to know. So if your mom asks if you had junk food, you tell her the truth, but if she doesn't ask, don't just voluntarily tell her."

Sleeping Through The Wake Up Calls

I missed out on a fair bit of involvement with Emma because being hugely overweight brings many physical limitations. I will talk about that more later on in the book. It hurt me. I have a lot of regrets about not losing the weight to be more involved in Emma's life.

It bothered Emma that I was putting on weight for her entire life. In one of the early grades of school Emma was learning in health class about the heart and what heart attacks were about, contributors to poor cardio vascular health, etc.. Emma was so overwhelmed with the similarities between what she was hearing in class and my former lifestyle that she literally had a panic attack right in class. They had to call Penny to come and take her to the hospital.

That was obviously a very traumatic event for Emma, her mother and me. However, that did nothing to cause me to act. I kept putting on weight and I did a terrible job at looking after myself. I suppose I was aware of my disappointed career expectations, in Newfoundland, with school, with the job in Peterborough. I was also aware I was now hurting Emma. I was aware it hadn't worked out with her mom… but I wasn't doing anything to change my circumstances.

There was another event that should have been a huge wake-up call for me, what should have been another shock into reality, but I guess I was too self-absorbed to notice. I must have been deeply entrenched in my own selfishness. I was lying to myself about my weight and lying to myself about not losing weight. Ultimately I just missed this wake-up call too.

I had a buddy who worked with me at Suncor by the name of Corey Carlson. What a great guy! He had a wife and two children. His passing was very unexpected. I remember the night of the accident which ultimately led to his death a few weeks later. We got off work that morning and we were just starting to be off for six days. He was wondering if he was going to do overtime that first night off. The night before, he was talking to me about it. He even asked me, "Ahhhh Bussey! Should I do overtime, or should I go hunting?"

He eventually decided to go hunting, so I came in to work

that next night and picked up the overtime shift. I was next in line to get the extra hours. I was glad for him to be off hunting and glad for me to make the extra money. The very next morning, as I woke up, my phone was vibrating with text after text after text, "What happened to Corey? What's going on with Corey? This is unbelievable!…"

While he was away that first night hunting he was on a boat with some buddies and when they went off to sleep down below, there was an issue with the heater and Corey suffered from Carbon Monoxide poisoning. I think it was about three weeks he was in the hospital in Edmonton, in rough shape. He was gone shortly after that. He just finally passed away one evening after hanging on for a few weeks.

He wasn't a very religious guy, or church-going, but they had his funeral in the Gospel Church in Fort McMurray, because it was the biggest church in town. The church was absolutely packed; standing room only. People came out of the woodwork for that funeral. When somebody passes away at 43 and leaves a wife and two kids behind, that touches a lot of people.

I grieved. I was very sad to lose my friend. I thought about it a lot. For some unknown reason though, even though I had thought about how fragile life is, how careful we need to be, how you never know when your time is — for some reason I still did nothing about it. I didn't apply the lessons from this situation to my life and start to get my butt in gear right then and there. I should have. The time lost with Emma should have been a wake up call. I don't know why it wasn't. It just wasn't. If anything, that love for my daughter, the one I love more than life, you'd think that alone would have been enough to make me say, "It's time to change!"

Any one of these major life events in and of itself could have been sufficient motivation to get me to lose weight. My daughter having a panic attack, afraid for my health, you would think that would be enough to motivate me. My good friend passing away in a tragic accident, you'd think that would be enough to remind me how short life is and motivate me, but none of it did.

Looking back I think, *the fire* finally did it for me, for some reason, that was the straw that broke the proverbial camels' back. All those motivators before should have been enough to do it for me, but they never did. To this day, I don't know why. I wonder about it sometimes, with the fire, how it all played out. It wasn't just a moment in time looking at some seats in a plane or on a bus. It represented years of misery, hurting myself and hurting others. I finally had enough and finally started to do something about it. Before that, I just kept rolling along, oblivious to it all.

I bought my condo in May of 2014, two years before the fire. Moving in I quickly settled further into a lifestyle that was comfortable but miserable. I liked my own space and I now owned a lovely new home to wallow in my misery on my own. I will unpack this more in future chapters, but suffice to say, it's not easy being close to 600 pounds. It's lonely. It's sad. It's painful. It's the rut I was stuck in and I was heading towards a slow death.

4

Packing On the Weight

Getting up to almost 600 pounds requires an *amazing* amount of living out of bounds. I had to eat a huge amount of calories and spend a lot of time on the couch to get my weight that high. It doesn't come naturally to keep the overeating routine up for almost two decades like I did. Between the time I got to Fort McMurray and the time of the fires, I had averaged putting on close to twenty pounds, *every single year*. It wasn't just the occasional weekend binge, or a box of donuts once or twice, it took years of feeling totally lousy and doing nothing positive to help myself out.

If I can be honest, I used to feel terrible about myself. There was this downward spiral of negative emotions that I was fighting a lot of the time. I think a big part of it had to do with the loneliness of living almost 6000 kilometres from home, not married, no girlfriend, no family close by; not quite hopeless, but close. I got thinking about being discouraged, disappointed, sad, frustrated, bored and fed up. The odd thing is, I'm a pretty positive guy who loves to laugh and have fun.

As I mentioned, I had lost some weight in college, but I had no idea how to keep it off. I hadn't adjusted my lifestyle and I put that weight back on. When I had first moved to Fort McMurray I was tipping the scales between 340 and 350 pounds.

I suppose I always knew I was overweight, but after being in Fort McMurray for five years, back in 2004 I really noticed I was getting "too" big. I had just come from my first visit back home to Newfoundland in five years. I had last been home in 1999, then I drove home in 2004. I had extra weight on then. I knew it, and it was a lot of weight, but nothing compared to what I ended up being. When I came back from that trip, after a full week on the road, eating in restaurants, staying in hotels, then great food back home, I got back on the road for the week-long trip eating in restaurants and staying in hotels again. When I arrived back in Fort McMurray, nothing fit. When I went back to work, I couldn't even do up my work coveralls any longer. Coveralls I wore just a month ago, I could no longer close. Those were size 2XL or 3XL.

Suncor provided all of our work coveralls. At the time, I think those were the biggest they had, 2XL or 3XL. I noticed my clothes were a whole lot tighter. I remember thinking when I was home for that visit that I had no discipline. Mom would cook up a beautiful delicious supper for me. I would eat the whole supper. I'd follow up with a piece of pie, a piece of cake, or whatever cookies she would have there. I would sit and talk with her, and then I would drive up to St. Anthony, a nearby town and go have fast food two hours after, like fried chicken. Not just a little evening snack, but I'd have another whole meal!

At home in Newfoundland, they have something awesome. It's fries, hamburger meat, cheese and gravy. Some folks call it the "Newfie poutine." They layer the fries with the cheese, then more French Fries, more cheese. Then they fry up the hamburger meat and put it on top of that, then more cheese.

Then I had three pieces of deep-fried chicken along with it. I had this *after* supper, a second meal before bed!

When I had the box of Newfie Poutine, the box would bend in my hand. The grease would be coming through the box. After I ate that I would go get a bag of chips and a couple ice creams on the way home. This was after a full meal at home! I knew I was out of control. I didn't really care. I told myself I would just do it for a while and then diet.

That's when my weight seemed like it really took off, it skyrocketed. I remember mom would even say, "You're not eating again after that are you? Why are you eating again?"

I had never been like that before, not to that extent, and I didn't know why exactly. When I came to Fort McMurray after the visit to Newfoundland, I noticed that was when I lost all discipline and to be honest, I had noticed on the road trip across Canada, I was eating all kinds of junk food on the road, sitting in my car, munching away. After that it seemed like from then on my weight just gradually and steadily went up. I finally weighed myself in January of 2016, and I was 567 pounds. I likely put on more weight in the next four months before the fire. I may have been closer to 600 pounds, but the last measured weight I had where I had actually stepped on the scales was 567 pounds. The numbers I share are not inflated in any way. I say 567 pounds because that's the real number that I know for sure, *conservatively*! That's the heaviest weight I ever saw on the scale, but I probably got even higher. I'll never know for sure because I didn't step on that industrial scale at work again before the fires in May, 2016.

I would look at myself those days and I knew I was big, but I had never imagined that I would get close to 600 pounds. I remember a couple friends and I were trying to guess my weight and one friend said, "You're definitely 600 pounds." I used to watch wrestling, and I was thinking, "Man am I actually bigger than Andre the Giant? Not height wise obviously, but weight wise?" I probably was. I was massive.

I reached a point where I just didn't care anymore. I was dealing with all the normal stuff in life. I was alone, single, feeling unwanted and undesired. I was dealing with everything in life by myself, with my family back east. By this time my daughter had moved down south to Red Deer. Birthdays and Christmas would come and go and I was alone, except for work and friends. I would eat because I was down. I was depressed, and then I'd be more depressed because I would eat. It was a vicious circle, a depressing cycle.

I lived by myself and I had no accountability, no positive peer pressure, it was all on me and I didn't care, so there was absolutely no discipline on my part. Not a bit!

I was making good money, I had a good job. I could afford whatever I wanted and didn't really have to keep an eye on my grocery budget. I could just go for it. I didn't drink or smoke, and I didn't do any drugs or have any hobbies or habits, so I could go out and buy whatever food I wanted.

Every day, especially when I lived by myself, I would reason with myself, "Why would I take all the time to go cook food for one person when I can just jump in my car and grab take out? There's my supper plan!"

I'd go to McDonald's for two Double Big Mac's, large fries, ice cream, pop. Or I could go to A&W, Burger King, Mary Brown's Fried Chicken, KFC every single day. They even got to know me at KFC. "We haven't seen you in a couple days. Where have you been?"

That's when I started to think, "Oh, maybe I have a problem here," but I managed to ignore those thoughts.

THE FOOD and the feeling of joy I would get as I ate it, was definitely like a drug. When my clothes started to *not* fit any longer, then I'd become more depressed, so I'd eat more to feel better. To me, I always felt good when I'd go to the grocery store and I had my fridge right full of junk food, then I'd feel happy. I felt a sense of success, because I didn't have to go out and embarrass myself to get more junk food. I had all this *happy feeling* food, right there in my fridge. Mission accomplished. I had a supply of good feelings in the privacy of my unaccountable home.

I could eat my junk food in secret which is a big deal to an obese person. Sometimes I felt like I could hide it, because looking in the mirror I didn't really see myself, how big I actually was (because I didn't fit in the mirror frame). I would convince myself that maybe other people didn't think I was *that* big either.

I'd sit on my couch and eat all this food, and I'd imagine I was not putting on any weight (because I wasn't weighing myself often). I'd eat it all in secret, at home or in my car. I'd live every day and convince myself that I looked fairly normal, or at least I looked no bigger than I did a month ago, but in reality I was gradually getting bigger, and deep down I knew it. I would try to get into friends' vehicles and I wouldn't fit. If I could get in, I wouldn't be able to put the seatbelt on. They would offer to come pick me up if we were going somewhere and someone would have to ask, "What vehicle are we gonna take?" because I wouldn't usually fit in any other ride except my own - and barely fit in that.

I was treating or rewarding myself non-stop. I had a good paying job, so why not? I didn't have to answer to a wife or a roommate. I was getting away with a totally undisciplined lifestyle, all the time. I was going to Tim Hortons, on a road trip, stopping for a coffee, but it wouldn't just be a coffee. I would get my usual, an extra large triple / triple and a couple donuts, and a big box of Timbits, and I'd sit in my car, stuffing my face while I was driving. (I will explain a triple / triple and Timbits shortly).

THOSE WERE the dog days of summer, because I was living like a dog, giving myself treats. For whatever reason, I kept up this charade for twelve years, from about 2004 to 2016.

I remember, even from 2001 to 2004 when I first started working for Suncor, my weight kind of stayed roughly the same, because I was always wearing the same sized pair of coveralls. I could fit into and operate whatever equipment I had to get into at work, but in 2004 the wheels came off the bus of discipline.

Breaking Through To Insanity — My own personal thought on what happens to people is this, "When you hit a certain weight, man, you have got to be careful." There's no science behind what I'm saying, it's just what I believe. For me personally, when I hit that certain weight and I came back from my trip to Newfoundland in 2004, it's like I just started running all the yellow lights, red lights too. I never weighed myself. I knew nothing fit, but I'd say I must have been 380-400 pounds. It was like those work coveralls were my last guideline of what was still within the realm of "normal", my last measurement. Once I broke that barrier, the sky was the limit. My weight kept going up from that point on.

At college, at least I was surrounded by a community, there was some social pressure, norms to follow. I mean, I would overeat then, but it was college, everyone was figuring out new boundaries and experimenting with their newly found independence. I didn't eat crazier than anyone else.

When I was in college and working my first few low paying jobs, I never had the funds to go nuts on food. In college I ate most meals at the cafeteria, I just ate what everybody else would eat. Sometimes, with the guys in the dorm we would order two-for-one pizza, so I had a little bit of excess. I've never been a big pizza fan, so I didn't stray far past my boundaries at school. However, in Fort McMurray, from 2004 and on I had the means, I had no boundaries, I had no girlfriend, no accountability — I was free to explode. Once I broke past the barrier of what work was providing, I was in that "special order" zone, for clothes, for seatbelts, for furniture, for everything. Once I stepped out of bounds, whether it's an inch out of bounds or a mile out of bounds, what's the difference, right? It's *all* out of bounds.

The breakup with Penny was hard. I'm not blaming her or making excuses, but at least when I was dating her for those few years, there was some accountability there. I still had to look somewhat respectable. It took me a couple years to get over her. It took a long time. With Emma still in my life, it was a continual reminder that I was alone, without Penny. I'm not saying that was the source of the problem, but it made me more aware of how far away the rest of my old friends and family really were.

Loneliness is a horrible feeling. The breakup was hard and I think that played a part in my overall feeling of being alone, so I would always go back to my safe thing, my happy thing, my treat, my reward, my comfort and that was food. No matter what, the weight gain was my own responsibility not anyone else's.

We often don't think, "I feel lousy, I gotta fix this." Instead, a lot of people abuse anything they can that makes them feel good; food, drugs, alcohol, and we never really address the lousy feelings themselves. We enjoy the feel good of food, and we don't think, "I feel lousy and I should get some counselling or talk to someone or get help."

We just think, "Boy, those Twinkies look great. That cake

looks awesome. That pie!" We just eat it and feel good for a moment.

The Old Morning Routine

Not only was I going through all of the negative emotions, but it seemed to always come back to the fact that I was going through it alone. I would wake up in the morning and I'd feel so hopeless. As soon as I woke up, I'd feel the negative feelings try to swamp me right away. As soon as I opened my eyes I'd remember how terrible my life was because every single area of my life was impacted. That first breath, I could feel the heaviness, the weight on my chest, my lungs, the laboured breathing. The simple act of getting out of bed reminded me of how big I actually was.

Bed — It was a fight, a physical struggle to get out of bed. I had a decent bed, but the mattress was on the floor because a bed frame wouldn't be able to hold my weight, it would eventually bend and break. The same with a box spring, it would crack if I had one under my mattress, so, I just had a mattress on the floor. My 567 pound weight on the mattress caused the mattress to sag in the middle. It was a banana bed. I wasn't getting a very good sleep either, because my body was so far from perfect, the way a 150 or 200 pound body should normally function with this mattress.

I would roll, literally roll to get out of bed. I would stand up and my legs would be all tingly from a lack of circulation from the weight squishing down on whatever part of my body that was on the mattress. I had to stand beside my bed to allow circulation to get moving through me once again.

Getting Ready — With great difficulty I would have to get ready for work. That was always a chore. For me, getting ready for work took much longer than the average, normal man. I would think, "This is not a bad dream, I am trapped in this. This is actually happening."

You would have thought I would have done something about it right away. Did I change? Did I say "Enough of this!"?

No. It kept getting progressively worse over the years. Every morning as soon as I woke I'd get pounded by these feelings, right away. I'd look for some relief, some type of happiness. I would go right to the fridge. I would eat cookies at 5:00 in the morning. I'd start the day with the breakfast of champions, Potato Chips and a Diet Pepsi. I'd eat whatever made me feel good, enjoying some breakfast and then getting on with my day. It would probably take me about an hour to get ready for work.

Good Bye Socks! —Putting my socks on was a struggle, to the point where I couldn't get them on anymore. I remember the last time I tried to put socks on. I tried for about twenty minutes to half an hour. It was impossible. I couldn't bend over because my gut was in the way. I couldn't lift my foot very high because my legs were so huge. I just couldn't get them up off the floor enough. I finally gave up. I just couldn't reach my feet to put my socks on any longer. Finally I was looking up at the clock and I figured, "I'm going to be late for work. I can't do this." I just left my socks. I shoved on my shoes. I was done with socks. That was a dark day.

Going without socks was bad in the summertime, but in the wintertime it was even worse. I had these thin little shoes with velcro straps. I'd wear the flimsy shoes with no socks while outside it was minus 40 in Fort McMurray. It would only take seconds for my toes to get freezing cold and they would stay cold most of the day.

Clothes — My gym pants were barely covering me, definitely not keeping me warm in the winter months. They were not very thick. There was nothing underneath those sweat pants, just my boxers. It's a wonder I didn't get frost bite in the winter months.

I would put on a shirt and this old winter jacket that was

size 6X. I have kept that coat, I still have it to this day. I couldn't do the zipper up because I couldn't close it around my big belly. People at work used to joke around with me and say, "Oh Bussey!" Everybody called me Bussey at work. "Oh Bussey, you're not very cold, you don't even have your jacket done up."

I would try to laugh it off, joking and say back to them, "Oh no, big guys don't get cold. All you guys are all skinny wimps. It's just *crispy* outside. It's not cold."

Really though, I was half frozen to death! I wished so badly that I could just fit into a normal winter coat, socks, winter boots and gloves. I never wore gloves or a hat because it kind of completed the *look* of open coat and velcro shoes to go without gloves or a hat.

Feeling Lousy — I felt like I couldn't do anything about it. There was no need to change immediately, so I'd just suck it up, basically, and deal with it. I would try to go on with my day, but I was miserable. I was discouraged. I was frustrated. I felt dead inside.

I desperately wished I was a regular, average-weight person. All I wanted was to be somebody that could get up in the morning and take a couple minutes to get dressed; who would only take a minute to put some socks on. I wished that I would be able to step out of my house and I could be one of thousands who slept normally, ate normally, dressed normally, got in a car, fit in a booth at a restaurant or used any bathroom. I wanted to *not be* singled out. I hated to go outside because I imagined people were staring at me. Everybody *was* staring at me when I was 600 pounds and I knew it. Just because I was big didn't mean that I was blind or stupid. I knew what was going on and I really wished to be normal again, to be honest.

My choice of self-abuse, my addiction, was a terrible choice, chronic overeating. One of the worst things about a food addiction that alcoholics and drug addicts don't have is that you just can't hide obesity like some other addictions. You can hide the early stages of sneaking food, a bag of Oreos stashed somewhere, a sneaky drive-thru visit on your own, but you can't hide being almost 600 pounds, or 300 hundred pounds for that matter. You can hide a six pack in the morning if you want; if you're good enough at it. You can even hide drugs to some degree. You can hide, you can go where there's people that aren't drug addicts, and you can blend in with regular people for the most part and no one might know. You can't hide being obese. I wore the shame of that all the time, a never-ending shame that I medicated with more and more good feeling, happy time junk food.

Tim Hortons Breakfast and Beyond

Where I work, they have these big buses that would drive around town and pick employees up at several bus stops. It's a wonderful benefit of working there. You can get on a nice, warm coach bus. You don't have to worry about the roads or the weather. I would spill into the next seat; I didn't just fit in one bus seat. Being pretty self-conscious of that, I chose to drive to work instead, then I didn't have to worry any more about fitting into the bus seat. I would have to get to work really early, because I always wanted to get a good parking spot, because I couldn't walk very far, another limitation of obesity.

On a work day I had a breakfast routine that I'd stick to very regularly. Every morning I would get the same thing at Tim Hortons. Tim Hortons is a massive Canadian coffee and donut franchise named after an iconic hockey player from the 60's and 70's. Tim Horton died in a car accident in the late years of his hockey career. In his last years he linked his name to the branding of a donut and coffee shop with businessman Ron Joyce. Horton's legacy lives on with over 3500 locations across Canada and over 850 more shops in 10 U.S. States.

I would get up in the morning and go to work knowing I was stopping at Tim Hortons. I would order two extra large triple/triples (three cream and three sugars). I would get a 10 pack of Timbits (aka "Donut holes" in America) and I would get an *Everything* flavoured bagel toasted, extra dark. I love them toasted right black, to the point where the Tim Hortons would fill up with smoke - that's how we would know it was cooked just right. That's the way I like them: crispy charcoal, with butter and herb and garlic cream cheese.

As I would drive off to work, I would drink one coffee on the drive. I would have my Timbits conveniently accessible on the passenger seat or in the middle of the car as a finger food and eat those as I would drive on my way to work. I would get to work plenty early. I'd have my second coffee and my bagel and catch the bus going down to the mine. Once I was on the work property, that's as far as I could go before having to take the bus the rest of the way.

That breakfast was probably about 2,200 calories. I could have eaten a lot more, but on work days that was my routine for reasons I will explain later.

Speaking of Tim Hortons, three years ago, I had a bit of a routine after my six days working were finished. My first day off work, I'd get off of night shift at 8 a.m and on my way home I'd stop at Tim Hortons. I would get my usual, an extra large coffee, triple/triple. I would also get a six pack of donuts and then I would usually get a breakfast sandwich or I would get some other sandwich. I would eat the sandwich, head home, have two or three donuts and then go to bed for five or six hours of sleep.

I would get up at 2:00 or 3:00 in the afternoon. Right away it would hit me, that I was obese. Those thoughts would hit me like a punch in the face as soon as I woke up, all the negative feelings of being that big would dawn on me. Those few hours of sleep an escape. They were an escape from my sad reality.

The only thing that made me happy, going off to sleep or waking up again, was knowing that I had donuts waiting for me on the table. It was something to get me out of bed. That was my motivation to start the day. That was all I looked forward to in the day, whatever food I could get inside of me to make me feel better.

The Messed-Up Menu

As embarrassing as it is I would like to share with you all of my favourite foods during those 14 years when weight exploded. I'm hoping you can get an accurate glimpse of how messed up, how excessive my eating was. This is NOT so that you'll say, "Tony was really extreme, I'm not that bad," and NOT so that I'll make you hungry talking about all my old favourite foods, but so that you might identify with me and say, "I might not be that extreme, but hey! Maybe I'm out of bounds too!" Whether it's an inch or a mile, out of bounds is out of bounds!

I'm not trying to speak negatively of the following foods. It's the opposite. I *loved* these foods and truth be told, I still do. However, anything delicious, especially the sugary stuff needs to be done in moderation, or in my case, I needed to completely walk away from these foods *permanently*.

Burger King — I love the Whopper, especially the Double Whopper. I liked going to Burger King because they had the Oreo cheesecake and the Hershey Sundae Pie that I enjoyed for dessert and I'd get fries and a drink obviously.

McDonald's — I'd usually get the Double Big Mac. Actually, I'd get two of those, that's 700 calories in each burger alone, plus an order of fries and a drink.

A&W — I'd always ask for a five-piece, even though they only had a three piece Chubby Chicken Dinner on the menu, I would ask them to add an extra two pieces for me, hot and fresh. On top of that custom five-piece Chubby Chicken Dinner I would get a couple orders of onion rings, or French

Fries, whatever I felt like and a couple of their famous root beers. After ordering that from the drive-thru I would sit in the parking lot and I would eat it all right on the spot. Then, I'd drive over to Tim Hortons and I'd get an extra large Triple-Triple and two or three doughnuts. Then, I'd go for a drive.

Mac's — On the way home, I would stop at Mac's Convenience Store and get a large bag of chips and a couple of ice cream novelties. I really enjoyed those ice cream sandwiches, two or three of those. The chicken dinner from A&W, the Hortons run and Mac's stop was easily accomplished in two hours.

That would be a good ending to a dayshift- after work meal and snacks. Then, I'd go to bed. I'd roll out of bed in the morning and have a big breakfast. Hopefully I'd have some junk food left in the fridge and I'd eat that too.

Mary Brown's — I love Mary Brown's fried chicken. I would usually get a five or six piece box of chicken there as well. I'd get their taters with it on the side.

KFC — I would usually get a four piece chicken dinner with fries and a Pepsi or something to drink. My appetite and portion size for KFC grew over the years.

One time my friend Corey, that passed away, was working a night shift to cover for me. The boys at work still talk about this funny story: He was working night shift, doing a mutual for me. He would cover my shift for me and I could cover his shift for him another day, where we would switch shifts basically. He didn't know, but I got him to work for me on the night of the time change one fall, when the clocks turned back an hour.

I didn't tell him what was happening. I just got him to sign the paper. He came to work, I was off. When he got to work that night, about an hour into his shift, he realized the time change was that night and that he was about to work a 13-hour long shift. He called my cell phone and hollered , "Bussey!You ****** ****** **** ***hole!"

He was laughing and swearing and he yelled, "You tricked me!"

He kept laughing then he said, "Well, you'd better bring me some chicken, Bussey! You'd better make up for this!"

I was relaxing at home, so I said, "Yeah, okay Corey. I'll bring you some chicken, Buddy," and I went to KFC.

He said he was tricked and that he wanted some make-up chicken and he swore a blue streak to make his point. That was Corey. I was laughing and he was laughing so I thought I'd do it - get him some chicken right away as a joke, kind of.

I went to KFC and I picked up a big bucket of chicken. I started driving out towards the work site. On the way out to work, the chicken smelled really good. It was practically jumping off the passenger seat at me so I took the top off the bucket and I started eating all the skin off the chicken — forty minute drive, smelling all eleven herbs and spices — why wouldn't I eat all that skin? I got out to the mine and he met me at the security gate. He laughed and grabbed the bucket of chicken, gave me a hug and said, "Thanks Bussey, you didn't have to do that, I was just kidding around, but I appreciate it."

He leaned forward toward me again and said, "Thanks for getting me to work this extra long night!"

"Oh, no problem, have fun," I replied.

When he got down to the mine, he opened up the bucket of chicken and realized the skin was eaten off half the chicken in the bucket. He called me up again, started swearing at me, but he laughed even harder this time. He said, "I should have known better." He and the guys at work talked about that for years afterwards.

At KFC in my early days of overeating I was getting a three or four piece dinner for a meal. I ended up getting a whole bucket just for myself when I was really overdoing it. At KFC and other restaurants, I was ordering normal combos that were fattening enough and then as time went on, I'd get two or even three meal combos. I was eating way too extreme at every restaurant. It seemed like I couldn't get enough. I couldn't satisfy the craving. No portion was enough. There was no feeling "full" or "satisfied."

Sometimes I'd get a meal and a couple of hours later, I'd be off for more fast food, or Tim Hortons, or a dessert portion that would feed four or five people. It was just like being a heroin addict, just constantly wanting the fix and then wanting more.

Every day was horrible. It's a good thing I didn't smoke or drink at that level of excess because I'd be a goner. The skin on my face was starting to turn brown. My eyes were getting ugly looking dark circles under them.

ICE CREAM AND PIES — I had a big weakness for ice cream. I loved ice cream. Dairy Queen ice cream cones were a favourite. I used to love going to Dairy Queen to get an ice cream cone; not chocolate dipped or any topping, just a soft-serve ice cream cone. I loved Häagen Dazs tubs of ice cream, cookie dough. Drumstick Caramel ice cream cones; I'd buy those boxes of four all for myself; I loved pie with ice cream; warmed up apple pie…Mmmm. Pecan pie, with some ice cream on it; I could sit down and eat the whole pie. Coconut cream pie was also a favourite. Some cake, I didn't buy a lot of cake, but every once in a while I'd enjoy a cake. For my birthday, I would go get an ice cream cake. I remember one year I went to Marble Slab Creamery and bought one of those huge cookie dough ice cream cakes. I ate that whole thing. I did that three different times. I would eat that for breakfast, dinner, supper. I'd get up in the morning and for breakfast I'd have ice cream cake. Oh, that was good. It probably had about 28 million calories, but it was delicious.

Potato Chips — I loved the chips, sour cream and onion chips, all-dressed chips, any kind of chips really. Those old school, onion ring chips; I used to love those things. I'd have some chip dip, drench those in dip and just indulge. It was nothing to sit down and eat a big bag, maybe two bags of chips. I never did develop a taste for the dill pickle flavoured potato chips though.

Chocolate Bars and More — O'Henry chocolate bars, I loved those things. Anything with peanut butter in it, like those Reese's peanut butter cups; all of those are delicious. I ate a lot of that, a lot of chips, a lot of ice cream, not much candy, but a lot of chips and ice cream. In general, I ate a lot of junk food.

Cookies — I loved cookies. There was this restaurant in Fort McMurray called Mrs. B's; Newfies owned it I believe. They had a section where it was all Old Maid pies and Old Maid cookies and all the traditional Newfoundland desserts.

Speaking of cookies, there was one style of cookie that I used to love; Mediterranean cookies. I found them in a little pack in the bakery at Sobey's grocery store. They had a variety of cookies in this pack and they were very sweet, delicious little things.

I also loved Oreo cookies. There's a guy at work, he used to bring Oreo cookies to snack on and somebody played a prank on him one day. They stole his Oreo cookies, they took out that middle white stuffing and they refilled it with minty white toothpaste. He was eating his cookies and it was toothpaste in the middle. That was a good gag.

Almost a cookie, but actually a "square", Nanaimo bars — a delicacy from the west coast of Canada — I loved those things.

Back Home Dessert — Mom would make all kinds of delicious peanut butter balls and traditional cookies. My favourite dessert dish of all time, I'm not entirely sure of the name of it, but it was "pistachio pudding pie" I think. It had a graham wafer base. Every time I'd go back home, my aunt would make me a dish of that scrumptious fare. I probably had the whole pan gone without any help.

Anything Deep-Fried — I loved it all, deep-fried chicken, French Fries. I loved chicken wings, especially those deep-fried chicken wings from Pizza 73. I used to eat a lot of KFC, Mary Brown's, a lot of burgers and all the greasy deep-fried sides.

Donuts — Any donuts that were cream-filled, I loved those things, especially in hockey season, I'd love to get those special Stanley Cup donuts. Maybe you remember Oreo donuts at Tim Hortons? I'd buy those things like they were going out of style — and they were — limited edition. I ate a lot of high sugar stuff.

Day Off Breakfast — I've shared my old morning routine of 2200 calories on a work day, but if I had a day off I would just binge, go crazy every day and any day on food. I would get up in the morning and for breakfast there were a couple of things I would make.

For one big breakfast I'd fry hash browns in a couple tablespoons of butter in the frying pan. Then I would add more butter to get them all nice and brown, so the hash browns were crispy and greasy. Next I would put four or five slices of processed cheese over them. Then I'd fry up a pound of bacon to have with them. I'd also fry three or four eggs. Finally I would add four or five slices of toast with that, all covered in butter. It's a wonder I didn't have a heart attack right on the spot eating like that!

The other calorie-heavy breakfast I would love to make was "fried egg salad sandwiches". Eggs themselves in a reasonable portion are a good, healthy and nutritious, especially poached or even hard boiled, but that's not how I used to eat them. I eat a lot of eggs now, but I used to make them in a very unhealthy way. I would fry up the eggs. Then I would add a lot of mayonnaise, cover them in mayonnaise really and put the toast on top. It tasted amazing.

I would have that for breakfast, get the kitchen cleaned up, then I'd go out for lunch. I'd usually go to Burger King or McDonald's and have the stuff I described above. Then I'd go to Tim Hortons, grab my usual extra large triple/triple and a couple of donuts. I'd drive around, maybe go down to the park and park my car by the lake somewhere. I wouldn't get out, just sit in my car, enjoy the view and chow down on my snacks.

More Fast Food — At supper time, I would go to KFC or Mary Brown's. It would more often than not be another fast food meal. Every once in while I would cook. Mostly, the only time I ever cooked at home was breakfast. I would get up the morning and I would have my coffee. For my coffee at home I'd buy a box of sugar cubes. I'd make myself a mug of coffee, put four or five sugar cubes in it and *then* add the French Vanilla creamer for added sweetener. I would have three or four cups of that and the big plate of breakfast. That was basically the only time I would cook at home. The rest of the day was mostly fast food.

Grocery Shopping — At the grocery store typically to start off, I would go to the pop aisle. If I found the cases of twenty-four of Diet Pepsi that was my preferred product delivery method — the two-four. A lot of times they didn't have the cases of twenty-four. They just had the little twelve-pack. I would prefer to buy three or four cases of two-four Diet Pepsi. Then I would get three or four bags of chips, a lot of times, sour cream and onion or all-dressed flavour. I'd go down the next aisle hunting for more junk food. I'd go through each aisle and I would get cookies and I would get chocolate bars and find little items I liked, "Oh, there's those cakes I like." I'd get cakes or bear paws, I'd load the cart right up. I'd just browse the inside aisles, never the outside aisles except the baked goods.

Next was the ice cream section. I'd get two or three tubs of Häagen Dazs ice cream, cookie dough was always my passion, and then put boxes of the Drumstick Caramel Cones, four packs like I said, in the cart. Sometimes I'd even get a big tub of ice cream and then just buy some ice cream cones on top of everything else, to make my own little cones at home. I remember there was this ice cream sandwich the grocery store had; a Reese's ice cream sandwich. Those had the big chunks of Reese's peanut butter cup in them. Those were so delicious that they were scary.

Then I'd keep going through the aisles. I'd get some eggs and bacon. I might buy some pork chops or a little bit of meat if I was feeling more ambitious, but usually nothing much healthy. In the end, it was mostly just junk food at the checkout.

That was my thing. When I went home and I unloaded my groceries, I'd say probably 80% of it was junk food. My entire fridge was full of junk. I had my cupboard full of cookies and snacks and I was relieved knowing I didn't have to go out in public anymore to get my fix. I was like a drug addict who went off and got enough coke supply to last him a week. I didn't have to go out and try to search for my next hit.

Going to a grocery store for me was a cause for anxiety *every single time*. It was painful, physically, to walk through a grocery store. Many times I would feel lower back pain and my feet would usually hurt a bit from walking. I'd *always* get people staring at me. Little kids pointed at me. I'd hear their little comments, looking at their Dad asking, "How come he's so big?"

It felt like there was a measure of judgement that followed me as I left the store. Everyone who looked into my grocery cart would see all the junk food; the cashier, the customer in the next aisle and the person bagging the groceries. I could almost feel the indignation.

I couldn't wait to get out of there, but I needed my stuff, my fix. I paid for it, rolled out of there and then when I got home I was okay. I'd talk myself through it, "I'm home now, I'm in my little safe spot. I can pig out all I want and nobody's here with the judging eyes. Nobody's here to get upset with me."

Other than the pop, *ALL* of those groceries would be gone in three days. When I woke up in the morning, and especially the next morning after grocery shopping, I was all set. I had endured the physical and more so the emotional difficulty and plowed past the anxiety so that my fortress of junk food, my stronghold of sugar was built again and I could hide away from the world, watch a movie, eat and escape.

In that old season of my life I would get up in the morning and I would *never* think about healthy eating. I would just think about all the junk food I had in my fridge. A lot of times in the morning, I would have two or three coffees with all that sugar and cream in it; right away I'd be looking at hundreds of calories even before I had a bite to eat! Sometimes I'd open up a bag of chips to start the day. Then I'd eat half a bag of cookies or some ice cream. Those were literally my morning breakfast "appetizers". Then after that I'd make some eggs and bacon and everything else I described.

Soda — Every day I would drink eight, nine or ten cans of pop. I always had a pop on the go, always had a cold pop in hand. That's part of the reason I didn't like to get a twelve-pack of soda. It would disappear too fast. A couple of years ago, I would literally go months without having a glass of water. Water consumption, even to this day, is still a weakness. I need to drink more water. I do drink more of it now, but then, it wouldn't be unheard of to go maybe even six months without a glass of water. I'd just be drinking coffee and pop. That'd be it. How did I survive?

I think that extreme pop and coffee intake might have been

part of the reason my skin was all turning brown. I used to get a lot of cuts and rashes up on my forehead where my skin was turning an unusual shade of brown. It would look like insect bites all over my forehead. I'm not entirely sure what happened but it started to disappear once I lost the weight. I don't have it anymore. Initially, I used to think maybe it was my hard hat, that the band inside my hard hat was cutting or scraping me. My doctor said a lot of times big people can suffer from malnutrition because we're not getting any of the proper nutrition, vitamins and minerals normally found in food-real food, like fruits and vegetables, the kind of nutrition that we need every day. I was huge and I could be eating all day long, but not getting any fruits or vegetables into me. I wouldn't buy any fruit. I'd hardly buy any vegetables. The only vegetable I'd get would be French Fries, maybe some onion rings if I felt like really upping my veggie game, maybe add a little bit of honey on that onion ring. I just didn't do veggies. It wasn't my thing. That's pretty scary when your healthy choice is, "I'm going to get some vegetables. I'll have some onion rings please!"

I never touched broccoli. The guys at work would mess with me and say, "Here Bussey! Have a piece of broccoli."

I'd say, "Ah. Little green trees, I don't want that. So disgusting."

Bathroom Restrictions — I didn't like eating much while I was at work. I would barely have anything other than breakfast, maybe some snacks. Partly, I was embarrassed about eating excessively in front of others, bags of chips and tons of junk food; I'd rather do that in private. The main reason I didn't eat much at work was that the bathrooms didn't fit me, I could barely get into a bathroom stall. I'm not trying to be gross, but if I had to go number-two at work, it was almost impossible because the bathroom stalls were too tiny for a 600-pound guy. If I really had to go to the bathroom badly I'd need to hike all the way over to the main complex. That was quite a walk for the 600-pound me. Today it's no problem. I can use any bathroom anywhere. During work time, in my heavy days I'd stick to the 2200 calorie 2 coffees, 10 Timbits and a bagel routine because that wouldn't fill me up too much and force me go to the bathroom. That high calorie, low-volume breakfast did the trick before work every day.

Helpful Friends — I have been very blessed with the friends I've had at work and people I have met in Fort McMurray. They looked past my discouragement, my weight, my pain that seemed to build over fourteen years. They saw me for who I really was. I worked with some of these people for years and they saw me gradually put on the weight over a decade and a half. They would try to talk to me about it and gently confront or challenge me to take better care of myself. I was stubborn. I would blow if off, "Ah, no, I'm okay. I'm good. I'm good."

Whenever I mentioned at work that I was going to try to lose some weight, they would all be very encouraging. They would say, maybe I should try to eat this or that; they would be really good about sharing little encouragements.

I had this one buddy at work, Anas Kabbaj, a really good friend of mine. He's from Morocco. We worked together quite a bit in the tire shop and became good friends. We're all good friends. There's a crew of eight of us on my shift. We're like a small family. We're all very tight. Anas and I have had a lot of heart-to-heart discussions over the years. We would sit together and he'd talk to me more than anybody else. He'd say things like, "You can't give up. You've got to keep trying. Don't quit."

Corey, my work friend that passed away would have a lot of talks as well. He used to be very concerned. Corey was very blunt, very outspoken, but he was a supportive peer. Corey would basically tell me to "F***ing smarten up!" He would swear at me, but I knew he really cared. He swore a lot, but he'd let me know he was very concerned that I wasn't going to wake up one morning. He would remind me that I had a daughter, so I should especially smarten up for her. He always had my back and would offer any help that I might need because it was tough to do that job being so overweight. He said he'd be there to help. Everybody offered to help. Even with Suncor, the company I work for, a manager approached me one day and offered me some help. The people at work were all incredibly supportive, but I still kept putting on weight! I had lots of friends that wanted to help but I didn't really have *ANY* accountability.

Getting By — I was too stubborn. I would sometimes see my size in the mirror. I saw all these clothes that didn't fit. I was well aware of activities I could no longer do, but I could still survive at the bare minimum every day. As long as I had that minimum survivability, still able to do some things on my own, I refused to get help.

Even though it was very hard, I could still to go to the grocery store. I could still barely fit in my car, so I could still go out. I could still wear shoes even if I didn't have socks, so, I could still walk just to get to my car, even though my feet were frozen. I could do the very minimum to get through my day. That was enough. I didn't need any help.

A lot of times supper was just pick up the phone and order food for delivery or take-out. I look back at all the money I spent. I wasted thousands of dollars on junk food. I'd order Chicken Wings or some other fast food right to my door. Typically, almost every day I would order or pick up some type of fast food.

Weight Loss Groups — During the years that I was putting on weight, I would try from time to time to do something to lose weight. There were weight loss groups that I would join for monetary rewards, which were substantial; one was five hundred dollars to join, with two or three thousand dollars to the winner. Whoever lost the most weight would take home the cash. Even that wouldn't be enough to motivate me to lose weight. Outside of all of that, beyond getting more money, I was trying to find some type of happiness. The only happiness I could find, at the time, was through food.

Late Night Eating — I used to eat a lot of junk food late at night. Late night food would just cause me all kinds of problems and really made me pack on the pounds.

As I said earlier, because of the bathroom situation, I didn't like eating much while I was at work, so, I would go all day and not eat very much. After work, I'd get home around 8:30 or 9:00 p.m., I would go to a fast food spot, and pig out before I'd go to bed. Being back in town, I was in my safe zone. I didn't care as much what strangers thought about me. At work I was limited and couldn't eat much, but then I'd get in my car and head to KFC, McDonalds, Mary Brown's Fried Chicken, Burger King or any other spot where I loved to binge. I'd eat a whole bag of chips or two bags in between stops. I look back on it now and it's just disgusting. It's no wonder the Bible warns us about gluttony. It was really and truly killing me, a slow death.

If I was home and I had no junk food in the fridge or cupboard, as lazy and unmotivated as I was, I'd be gone out the door in a second to get some unhealthy snacks immediately. I'd come back home afterwards and I would be very happy with my big bag of chips, a couple chocolate bars and some ice cream. I'd settle down on the couch watching TV, head off to bed and get up the next morning. I'd see the chip bags and all the empty containers on the coffee table and be disgusted and disappointed with myself. Five minutes later, I'd be looking for more junk food!

No Exercise — There was really no activity in my life, no physical fitness or exercise of any kind. There was a slight bit of movement at work where I was changing tires on huge mining machinery and vehicles, but a lot of that was machine work where I did very little except operate the machine. I would walk from my car to the door of work or home. I'd walk to the door of the restaurant or store — but I'd usually get drive-thru. I'd walk from my condo to the car; I'm talking a few minutes of walking a day, total! I was a full-blown couch potato. The most exercise I'd get in any given day was two or three minutes of walking just to get where I needed to go to survive and not a step more if I could help it.

Excuses — You don't get to that size by eating a little. People talk about, "I'm big boned!" Or people say, "It's hereditary." I've also heard, "It must be a thyroid issue." Let me be clear. For me, 600 pounds had nothing to do with being "big boned" or a hereditary problem or a thyroid issue. My weight was just about laziness, stubbornness and selfishness on my part. It was all about having no respect for myself, I simply didn't care. There must have been some mental or emotional things motivating me, I'm sure, because I never would have eaten that much if I was happy and well adjusted. I wouldn't have eaten that much if everything was going great in my life. It was a fix. Every time I ate I felt happy. Outside of that I was entirely miserable.

Man Made Junk — I think that many things that are man-made might give us temporary happiness but many of those things, especially too much of those things will eventually damage or kill us. Everything that God made or Mother Nature made, whatever you believe, none of those things are going to ruin me. The things that could destroy my life, smoking, alcohol, drugs and junk food have the potential to do some serious damage. All of those things, if you abuse them, or overdo it, are going to kill you. Man-made foods are dangerous. Prepared meals, salty and sugary foods can make people huge. Man-made food can push us into a whole world that's not designed for big people, which leads to a downward spiral of discouragement and depression.

Wingicide — I used to go to Pizza 73, a big pizza chain

in western Canada, where I'd order take out. I'd get 20 golden crispy chicken wings, a box of curly fries, two bags of bite-sized brownies and then have my diet pop from the fridge at home. After eating that I would lie on the couch for an hour-and-a-half, then drag my butt up off the couch, and walk to the convenience store (because they didn't do delivery). I would get a bag of chips, the big bag, some chip dip, three or four ice cream sandwiches, (those things alone were $5 each) I'd buy some chocolate, those chocolate covered almonds and take it all back to my condo. If I found those almonds at a convenience store, it was like I found a gold ticket. I'd pig out on those. The next day, it'd be more junk, more sugar, carbs and sweets. When I would eat like that I would enjoy my ten or fifteen minutes of feeling happy. As soon as I stopped eating the guilt would set in and I knew exactly what I was doing. I immediately felt miserable and knew I was slowly killing myself, putting myself out of my misery. I didn't want to die. I didn't want to kill myself. I didn't want to commit suicide, but I couldn't face tomorrow, so I would slowly kill myself with chicken wings and chocolate covered almonds.

Lies Upon Lies — I would lie to myself about all this and say, "I'm going to start eating healthy on Monday because I'm making a mess of my life and I feel awful." I was actually going to do it. I was going to start. I was going to move into a whole new lifestyle. Then to celebrate my new lifestyle change, I'd go get more junk food because it was only Thursday and if I was going to start on Monday, I only had three or four days to get whatever happy food I could get in me. Again, all weekend long I would stuff myself with empty calories. Now I was doubly happy, because I'd be eating all this junk food and on another level I was happy because I had convinced myself of the lie that I was going to start changing my lifestyle on Monday. It made me feel less guilty about eating all the junk food on the weekend. Then Monday would come, and nothing would change.

Working 12-hour shifts, I'd come home and my feet and legs were in pain. I was so depressed about being the size I was that I would open up the fridge and see a big friendly cheesecake sitting there. It was just me and my cherry topped friend, with no one to be accountable to, no one to look over my shoulder. I could eat as much as I wanted. Before I knew it the fridge would be empty, my belly would be full and I'd have a couple minutes of shallow happiness.

That cheesecake was my comfort. Two tubs of ice cream in the freezer and boxes of ice cream novelties were my happiness drug. When I ate, there were no problems, but in the back of my head I knew, "I shouldn't be doing this. I'm killing myself. This is the whole reason I'm miserable."

To try to get that weight off was such a huge challenge, that I never thought I'd ever be able to do it. I had never truly tried. I knew if I ate that junk food, for that brief moment, I would forget feeling miserable. Junk food was my girlfriend, my family, my problem-free-zone and my drug. It was everything to me. I wouldn't be in the house without having it. If I didn't have it, there was a convenience store right behind my home that I would rush to visit.

Looking back on the money I spent on that habit is unbelievable. I look back on all that now with a sense of wonder. Who was that guy? How could I have been that out-of-control?

I was out of control with what and when I would eat. I can't describe it. It was a "constant craving" as the song says, I was always wanting something more. It didn't matter if I looked happy, I was continually miserable. I was often upset inside, frequently depressed, very discouraged and down on myself because of my weight. That's why I know I will never go to that lifestyle again. Now that I have all that weight gone every-day-living offers me newfound joy. I will never pack on weight like that again. The humiliation of seeing the empty seats beside me on the bus and on the plane were the moments in time that finally ended ***the lie***. I will never again get sucked into the temporary insanity of choosing a short-lived taste in my mouth or warmth in my belly that was there for an instant, but then quietly and slowly killing me.

What a rip-off. What a lie.

5

What It's Like Being Clinically Obese

The world is not built for 567-pound people. Being huge is something that most people cannot relate to very well. Until you have an extreme addiction like I did, you can't really imagine how this kind of problem impacts your life every single day, often many, many times each day. Why *would* you want to imagine that? I don't mean to be unpleasant or gross in any way, but let me briefly paint a picture of how radically messed up my life was just over two short years ago:

Carrying Extra Weight — I spent about a decade in what I would consider the obese category. I was overweight for twenty years or more, but I was over 350 pounds for fourteen years. Putting on those twenty or so pounds a year was like lying in a torture cage or a stretching-rack in a dungeon. It was painful, but it was self-inflicted agony. Eventually I found myself almost 350-pounds overweight. I had a friend ask me what it was like. This picture emerged: Imagine taking one of those blue water jugs that you take on a camping trip, or one of those big, clear plastic water jugs they sell at the front of the grocery store, or a specialty water store - those are fifty pounds each. Imagine taking seven of those water jugs and tying them to your back, all seven jugs. Imagine 350 extra pounds and then going for a five minute stroll down by the lake! That's what I mean by "torturous."

It was *not* easy. I get emotional thinking about all the extra weight I carried for so long. It nearly killed me. Even walking was nearly impossible. I'd walk across a street, or even a few steps and I would have to stop to take a breath. There'd be many nights I'd go to bed early because I'd just be tired out. I was always exhausted.

Mornings — Sometimes I'd pray I wouldn't wake up in the morning, totally despairing and frustrated with how much my life sucked. I wasn't suicidal, just very discouraged, not wanting another day of this horrible pain. What I had to face the next morning, every morning was unbearable. I loved life. I still do. Life is beautiful. Even during those dark days, there were still positive aspects about life. Every night I knew what I was going to have to face the next morning. I was losing my ability to handle facing that with a positive outlook.

Being obese was a self-imposed handicap that had put me in my own prison. It was the end of everything normal. That heaviness of heart, that unbearable feeling was there every day. When Corey passed away, for whatever reason, it still didn't change anything. Friends talking to encourage or challenge me didn't change anything. My daughter breaking down in school because she was afraid I was going to have a heart attack didn't change anything. Seeing the physical effects on my body didn't change anything. The loneliness didn't change anything. For whatever reason, none of that changed a single thing.

We're talking over 4,000 mornings of frustration where I would have woken up in my banana-shaped-bed, sore, pins and needles, headaches, discouraged with very low energy. Those years were very tough. I really went through the grinder not caring about myself, not caring about the things I had or who I was hurting.

Could I Just Be Normal? — In many, many areas of my life I stood out like a sore thumb. My one deepest, secret desire was to just be normal.

I longed just to be one of thousands, a regular Joe that kids would pass in the grocery store and not notice, not even look at because they just blended into the crowd. I longed for that. After years of being huge, I hated going anywhere. I'd come home from work and I'd just stay in my condo. I spent a lot of time by myself. Which was making a bad situation even worse.

The Medical Parts

Pancreatitis — Thankfully I haven't had any of the problems often associated with obesity. I haven't had any real knee problems. I was starting to get some lower back problems just before I began losing the weight. I was also having some foot problems.

In 2017 I had to have my gall bladder taken out after I'd lost much of the weight. I asked the nurses about some of the details as I recovered. They told me that with really big patients what happens, when people eat so much fatty food, the body is accustomed to taking that fat and dealing with it, getting rid of the bile. However, when I changed my diet and stopped eating as much fatty food, my body was still producing this bile. When that bile is not being used it turns into stones. That's where my gall stones came from, and that's what needed medical attention.

I ended up having pancreatitis. In the summer of 2017 when I had already lost a lot of weight I was in the hospital for almost two weeks in total as a result of being 350 pounds overweight. They flew me to Edmonton a couple times. I had a stone caught in my bowel duct. I asked about it afterwards, "What would have happened to me if I was still 600 pounds?"

One Doctor who was part of the medical team spoke to me

very openly. "We knew about your weight," she said, "Tony, you probably wouldn't even have been able to use the washroom here. We would not have been able to get a robe on you that would have fit. We wouldn't have been able to fit you into a regular wheel chair. You probably wouldn't have fit on a stretcher. It might not have supported your weight. If we had to fly you to Edmonton for further medical attention, we probably would have had to get a special plane to come in. If we couldn't get a plane we would have had to put you in a special ambulance all the way to Edmonton, or maybe even an ambulance all the way to Calgary because you would've had to go to a special room that deals with people your size."

Then she said, "On top of all of that, to put you under for surgery, to give you an anesthetic, would you even wake up from that? Could your heart take that? This is all just from a routine gall bladder procedure. It could have killed you, Tony!"

That's why they did an actual case study on me. There's a nursing textbook that's coming out in the near future, where the results of the case study will be published; the topic is how to train nurses to deal with obese patients. There were many other medical issues I had to deal with while I was still heavy.

Sleep Apnea and Acid Reflux — I used to snore severely and breathe so poorly that I couldn't get a sound and restful sleep. I also used to wake up in the middle of the night, choking. That doesn't happen anymore since I've lost weight. I used to wake up and have acid reflux coming up my throat. I couldn't breathe, it was like I was choking to death. It would settle down after I'd sit up, awake for a few minutes. I'd lie down and as I was falling back to sleep then I'd get that acid coming up and feel choked nearly to death all over again. What a terrible way to wake up in the middle of the night! I haven't had that issue in the years since I started losing weight.

The doctor wanted to send me for tests, for the sleep apnea and acid reflux when I was heavy, but I would never go for tests. Being that size, the last thing I wanted to do was go to a hospital or a lab or get tested for anything because I was always afraid they'd never let me leave again. They never had the right equipment to fit me. I couldn't even get something as simple as my blood pressure reading. They couldn't get the cuff around my arm.

Blood Pressure Cuff — The technicians would put the sleeve three quarters of the way around my arm and I'd have to do my best to hold it tight. I went to a doctor one time, and he couldn't read my blood pressure at all. He actually asked me to go to the drug store and buy my own blood pressure cuff. I said, "Yeah, okay. See you later, bud." I never went back there.

Later, there was a nurse that I was doing the case study with, studying obesity, she told me, "That's horrible, because, if they really want to test your blood pressure, they can take the cuff and wrap it around your forearm. The cuff doesn't have to be on your bicep. It's better to read from the bicep, but not mandatory. They should know that." It was all just a part of the medical humiliation I went through being clinically obese.

Dental — I had to go to the dentist one time years ago. I had a bad tooth for a long time and the pain was intense. I was thinking they wouldn't be able to help me. How are they gonna work on a man my size at that little dental office? I hate taking any kind of pills, even pain relievers, but I was popping Tylenol, the pain was so bad, I was popping them like they were candy. I think I took five or six extra strength pills in one afternoon.

I was sitting in the parking lot of the dental office late in the afternoon arguing with myself whether I would go in or not. The pain was so bad that I finally figured, "Screw it, I gotta go upstairs to the dentist office and at least try to get help for this pain."

I went to the Morrison Dental Centre in Fort McMurray. They were great. I went in to the office, and the dentist looked at me. I figured I knew what he was thinking, something like, "How am I going to manage this big guy in here?"

They put me in the dental chair. I barely fit. I was spilling over the edges. The dentist said I was the first guy he ever had to work on where he had to stand up. Usually, he'd just sit on his stool and roll up beside the patient's head and work on his mouth. He couldn't get close enough navigating around my belly, my huge neck, shoulders and head. In the end he just stood up and bent over me to access my mouth. They weren't sure how much anesthetic to give me. I guess I was too heavy to be on a chart that probably didn't go up to 600 pounds.

That brave dentist went ahead with his team and they did the work, thank God. He took the tooth out and got me fixed up, but that's the reality of being obese. When you're big, you just can't count on the normal day-to-day things that we all take for granted. The world is just not designed for really big people. Charts can't handle it. Chairs can't handle it. Change rooms are too small. Bathrooms are too small. Nothing fits for the super huge man or woman.

The Medical Exam —They do a physical on us at work every couple years. They are really great at looking after their employees. One year, while I was doing my physical, I broke their scale. It wasn't one of those upright medical scales with the sliders on it. The scale was just a digital bathroom scale they had on the floor.

I stepped on it, and, I didn't know I had broken it at the time, but I heard about it a little later. A mechanic who was on the same shift as me went after my appointment to get his medical done. The nurse told him, "That the big guy broke the scale." That mechanic couldn't get his weight checked during his annual medical appointment thanks to me breaking the scale.

Dark Skin — If you look at photos of me during my last two years of being obese, you can see dark skin on my forehead, a brownish, blackish colour to my skin.

As I mentioned earlier, I was only drinking Diet Pepsi and coffee and I rarely drank water so that may have been some of the issue. I'll never know for sure.

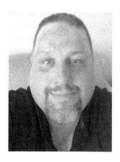

My darkened skin as my body was likely releasing toxins and I may have been malnourished.

Initially, they thought that the discolouration was dirt, but it didn't wash off. My doctor later told me that it was just "stuff" coming out of my skin. That's how I looked just a couple days before I started losing the weight. The picture above shows how my skin looked. I was totally stressed out in this photo, knowing I had to fly soon. I hated flying. I knew I wasn't going to fit in the plane flying back to work after the first evacuation.

Whatever garbage was in my body, it was just starting to come to the surface. This skin issue had been going on for a couple years, getting progressively worse. I talked to another doctor who told me that sometimes this happens to people that are really big. She told me that I may have actually been suffering from malnutrition.

My body was not getting the nutrients it required. All I was getting was greasy food and junk food, sugar and salt and empty calories. She told me it was likely that it was becoming harder for my heart to push the blood, oxygen and nutrients throughout my body. My blood was not exactly full of nutrients with my diet!

My skin was getting darker on the surface. My forehead looked like it was always dirty or that I had been sun tanning with a hat pulled half way down my forehead, but not in a straight line. My forehead really looked weird. I got the impression my body was ready to go on strike; it was giving me signs, sending me messages. It was saying, "You either shape up, or you're done!" My doctor didn't know for sure what the brown skin was about. I might never know for sure.

Dr. Robert Tomilson is a Doctor of Natural Medicine with the BIE Clinic in Oakville, Ontario. He is recognized as a leader and pioneer in his field in Canada. When the body is sending out warning signs, he is brilliant at connecting the dots to figure out what's going on. He has helped countless patients. Dr. Rob suggested several possibilities concerning the brown skin:

The dark skin might have been "liver spots," also called "age spots" which often show up in seniors but can manifest earlier too. With all the excess sugar and junk I was eating it is possible that there were localized concentrations of the brown pigment called lipofuscin, which accumulates throughout the body. Perhaps that was starting to show up on my face and especially my forehead.

It was also likely that the process of *glycation* was happening where all the sugar I was eating was bonding to protein molecules. That can cause all kinds of skin reactions including aging and discolouration. It can happen before people become diabetic, the pre-diabetic stage, a warning sign.

It also may have been caused from rancid fats under the skin. With my diet three years ago having lots of greasy and deep-fried foods and hardly ever any fruits or vegetables the body may have been storing those excess fats under the skin. Those deposits can turn rancid and cause swelling, inflammation, irritation or the manifestation of brown or red skin.

Lastly, it may have been a selenium deficiency caused by a lack of nutrients which can lead to skin changing shades or colour. Similar to what my doctor said about malnutrition.

When I stopped eating sugar and fat in May of 2016 Dr. Rob later suggested that my skin would have immediately cleared up for any of these possible situations listed above, especially the latter three issues. If he had he seen my brown skin three years ago to offer a diagnosis, his recommendation definitely would have been to remove fatty and deep-fried foods, white flour and sugar from my diet. I think that it's neat that even though I had limited knowledge of diet or fitness, common sense told me to cut out sugar, junk food and all the deep-fried fast food. It's not that I needed more education or more science, I just needed to do what was obvious, what was more natural. I think most of us know these obvious principals — cut out the sugar and junk and go for a walk. We might read a book thinking knowledge is power, but not always. It can help, but for me, the power to change was on an airplane, taking up two seats, realizing I was hurting people, in a terrible, selfish way.

Neck and Back Pain — I didn't look like I even had a neck. I had a lot of hanging skin around my neck. I was puffed right out. The back of my head looked like there were ten sausages rolling down my neck.

There was considerable back pain. Some days, I'd get home and my back would be hurting quite a bit. Although I didn't have as many back problems as one would have thought, there were days when my lower back would really bother me. I think I avoided a lot of issues losing weight when I did.

Eyes — For some reason, just before I started losing weight my eyes were a problem. One eye would be full of puss and my vision would become cloudy. I don't know what was causing it.

That was why I thought I might be getting diabetes. Between the tingling I was feeling in my legs in the morning and the issue with my eye, I thought for sure I had diabetes. I was checked out after I lost the weight and found I didn't have it. Maybe I did or I was heading that way, but I don't have diabetes now.

I would be at work, or at home and my one eye would start

clouding over. It would get all watery. Green discharge would be coming out of the corner of my eye. I would get water leaking from my eye and pouring down like tears. It was obviously not a good sign. My body was in trouble. You can see from the picture how dark my eyes were getting and the dark circles under my eyes but that all went away as I started losing weight.

The Day to Day Physical Limitations

Clothes — The last pair of jeans I owned were a size 66 inch waist and they didn't even fit me anymore. They were way too tight for me to wear to Corey's funeral. I did wear them for the funeral, but I barely got them on. After I grew out of those jeans all I could wear were size 7XL gym pants. I think I had three pairs of gym pants and that was it for my pants selection. My wardrobe was reduced to those sweat pants and some pretty ugly shirts. I would wear those gym pants everywhere, to work, at home and around town. It didn't matter if I was going to the movies or changing tires, that's all I had to wear. I had to be careful with them. The stores rarely had that size in stock.

I was up to a size 6XL shirt. I would always get shirts dirty and stained. When I was that big and trying to eat, my belly was in the way of everything I did. It was complicated to eat. I was always dropping and spilling food. I had stains on everything. Being able to perform the normal little day-to-day tasks that people take for granted, tasks like *eating without spilling* was an area that I longed for a level of being "normal" again.

I have realized since those days that once I crossed that "who cares" line and I let my body go, I really didn't care very much about *anything*. I had no pride in myself and I took pride in nothing, not my appearance or my things. I cared about nothing in my life. I'm a pretty clean person, but I'm a lot cleaner now than I was then; much tidier than I was then. Now

I take pride in having a shirt that doesn't look like a fraternity-house-rib-fest-stained-table-cloth.

My daughter lives down in Red Deer 600 kilometres south of Fort McMurray. When I would go down to visit her, I would go into the George Richards Big and Tall store. A lot of times I would shop there and they didn't have anything to fit me. The biggest shirt and gym pants they had in stock was usually a 5X. When I walked into a big and tall store and they didn't have clothes to fit me, that was *very* discouraging.

Not only are clothes harder to buy for big people, but the different styles and colours of clothes that are available for obese people are very limited. There are no materials that breathe easier, no products that are lighter weight. Those options are easily purchased for sizes S - XL, but you cannot find such options as a big person looking for 6XL or 7XL. The material is heavy, almost like it's made out of burlap or canvas. For thinner people, there are many clothing options like wearing khakis, or light and stretchy material, waterproof fabrics, hiking and walking friendly options. These possibilities didn't exist for me for 14 years of my life.

When I was over 500 pounds I'd go into a store and just say, "Oh, that fits? Okay I guess I'll take it."

It wouldn't matter the colour, it wouldn't matter what it looked like, I'd hardly notice or pay attention. My decision to buy came down to, "Well I can't go around naked, so that's what I have to buy!"

Even buying a belt was a huge ordeal. I had a "special" belt for the last time I could wear my pants, the size 66 jeans I wore to the funeral. I didn't have a belt at that time. I finally did find one, long after the funeral. Before that, I didn't have a belt for that would fit. I bought two belts and I spliced them together. Where I had them joined, I would keep the buckle hidden on my right side. I made sure the belt I bought was black and I wrapped the spliced buckle part in black electrical tape, so no one would notice it from the front. It *looked* normal. That was the goal, just to be normal.

Sitting, Walking, Falling, Bending — Sitting down was usually a relief for me, if I sat down carefully, safely and sitting a certain way. Many times as I sat down I would elevate my foot, just to take the strain off of it. It's tough carrying around the equivalent of seven water jugs all day long. Thankfully, I didn't have a lot of swelling and from what I've seen and known of obese people, that's one of several reasons why I think must have been a miracle I didn't have serious issues, or even death. To walk around carrying the equivalent of an extra person and a half on my back, day in and day out, for fourteen years is unbelievable. I waddled. I hadn't really walked for over a decade.

To go three years with no socks at all was amazing! There was really no swelling of any kind, in my feet or legs. I could not reach my feet to massage, rub or wash the bottoms of them. I hadn't seen the bottom of my feet in at least three years or more. I clearly remember getting out of bed in the morning and feeling tingling and numbness in my legs, having to stand by my mattress until the circulation got going again. The bottoms of my feet were sore from having no socks in my work boots. It was painful. There were a couple of times I came close to twisting my foot because of the way I was walking. That always scared me, because if I had twisted my foot on a rock or stepped on something uneven, I easily could have fallen down and broken my ankle, a leg, or my hip. Then what? Imagine what it would be like having a 600-pound man sitting on a couch with crutches for two months.

When I dropped anything, it was very hard to pick it up. I hated bending over with anybody around because it was embarrassing. The only way I could bend over would be to straddle my legs apart and kind of lean down. My stomach would be in the way so I would have to adjust to get around it and get my fingers near the floor. If I dropped a pen, I would try to kick it over to a spot where I had some room to flail around to get it. I hated dropping anything. A lot of times if I dropped something, the guys would be kind and help me out, "Oh hold on Bussey, I'll come get that for you."

All my friends, workmates, they were all very helpful, very sympathetic and supportive. They were very concerned. I found out after I lost the weight, how concerned they were. They used to talk about it with each other when I was heavy. They didn't know what to do. I feel bad for putting them through that, because they were genuinely concerned that I was going to drop dead one day. The struggle to pick things up is just another ugly reminder of how messed up and awkward my life was.

Driving and Parking — It was hard to find a bathroom to use, if I was traveling out of town. Not a lot of facilities would fit me, their bathrooms were tiny. Consequently, I didn't venture out too much. When I would drive somewhere locally, whether it was the grocery store, the mall, a restaurant or anywhere I had to park my vehicle, parking was an issue. Best case scenario, I would try to park next to a handicapped spot backed in so my door would open towards the disabled spot. I didn't have a handicapped permit, so I wouldn't park in the handicapped spots, but I really needed extra space to get in and out of my car.

This is something normal sized people wouldn't worry about or think about. The typical handicapped spaces are much wider. If I parked my drivers-side door next to the handicapped space, I didn't have to worry about anybody parking too closely next to me. Otherwise, if I was in a regular parking spot and somebody parked too close to my vehicle, when I came out of the store I would have a lot of trouble getting in the drivers side. I wouldn't be able to squeeze in. If I could park next to a handicapped space then I knew that even if somebody who was handicapped came in, they would have to leave enough room to get out of their vehicle, so I would have enough room to get into mine. I was essentially handicapped.

There were a couple times when I got to my car in a parking lot and I could *not* fit into it because another car was parked fairly normally, but a little too close beside me. Those times I had to approach a complete stranger and wave them down to request help. Totally embarrassed I would give them the keys to my vehicle and ask, "can you move my car out for me please, I don't have enough room to get in."

People were very helpful. One good Samaritan even got mad at the person who had me blocked in. He ranted, "those idiots, how can people be so inconsiderate!" He got in my car, backed it out for me and handed me the keys. I was very humiliated.

Parking at the end of a row or near the handicapped spots, those were little techniques, little tricks I had to learn to survive. It was bizarre how I needed to live to get through those simple day-to-day tasks. To this day, when I park somewhere, those old habits still kick in. I'll park next to a handicapped space. After doing it for fourteen years old habits die hard.

The Seasons — Winters I was frozen, summers I was really hot. I couldn't be comfortable at all when I was *Tony the Large*. My favourite time of year was probably the spring. It wasn't too hot, it wasn't too cold. It was the time of year farthest away from facing another winter again. In the summer I would drip sweat like a waterfall. I'd be so hot in the summer, that the sweat would just drip off my nose even if I wasn't doing any physical activity. I would step out of my car and break a sweat just walking ten steps. I tried to stay in the shade and air conditioned places as much as possible.

Photos — When I was the large size, I hated getting pictures taken. I rarely took a selfie. I hated when someone would say, "Smile!" and try to take a picture of me. That's why you will notice that there are not many photos of me on my social media from that era; some, but not many. My social media page was starving for uploads back then.

Movies — When I was at my biggest, as I said earlier, it would impact every area of my life. I remember I would take Emma to the movies and she couldn't even sit in the seat next to me at the theatre. If I did sit next to her, I'd spill over into her seat. She would sit one seat away from me leaving a vacant seat between us.

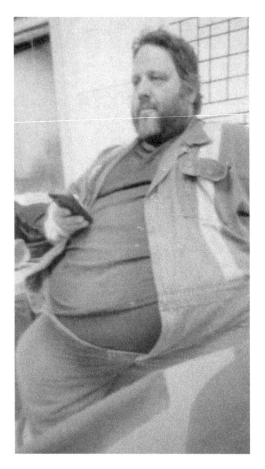

My "before" photo.

Car — It seemed all I did in life was eat, drive, sleep, work and watch TV. One of my big and somewhat safe adventures was going out for a drive. I'd pull into a drive-thru to order some fast food. I'd go for a little drive, grab more fast food and go for another drive. Even that was complicated, because I could barely fit in the car. Sitting in the car, my seat was pushed all the way back, jacked right down to the floor. I had a seat raising and lowering option in the front seats so getting the seat as low as it would go helped with headroom.

I always opened the sunroof cover to give me an extra couple inches of head clearance, but I'd still be squeezed right in there. I would be elevated several inches higher than a regular-sized person because I was carrying many extra pounds all over my backside. My head was usually rubbing up against the ceiling so having the sunroof cover open would give me that last little bit of head space I needed. The sunroof would be closed, but the cover would be slid back to help me.

My left arm would be wedged up against the door because it was twice the size of a normal arm and my belly pushed it even further left. The steering wheel would be touching my gut in front. At work or home, sitting in a regular chair my gut would come right out to my knees almost, a couple inches away from my kneecaps. That's how far out my gut would be sticking out. Seated, I could barely see my legs, my thighs were 90% covered by belly fat. That didn't leave much room for a steering wheel in front of me.

Getting into a car when you are carrying around weight equivalent to two average-sized washing machines is difficult. When I was sitting in the car, it would look like I was seven feet tall. Sitting in my car, that extra four or five inches of fat on my under-carriage made me look like a giant. I would get out of the car and just be a regular height of 5'9".

I used to have a Dodge 300 that was big enough for me even when I put on all of the extra weight. I was taking Emma to the movies in Red Deer a few years back and my car broke down, permanently. It was an older car, high mileage, having a lot of problems with the steering and some other issues that made it not worth repairing. I went to the dealership, and they asked what I wanted. I said, "Well, I'm kind of limited here." I said, "Bring me over another 300 to check out."

They brought a beautiful, almost new, maybe a one-year-old Chrysler 300. I love those cars. I went to get into that car, and I couldn't fit. I don't know if they made the newer ones a little smaller, or if I had just stretched the old one I had, but that was very shocking to me. Here's this huge car right in front of me, one of the biggest cars that anyone can buy, and now I couldn't even wedge myself into it. It was not just clothing stores that were embarrassing and humiliating, now buying a vehicle had become difficult too! This was all getting even more embarrassing to me.

I was at a dealership telling a sales guy that I can't fit in any of the vehicles that he had in stock. Dodge cars, come on man, they're *big* vehicles. Next he brought over a Dodge Charger and he said, "Try this one. We make 'em a bit wider for cops." They were being polite to me, but I think I knew what they were thinking. I'd always suspect what people were thinking in their heads, thoughts like, "Oh my goodness, this guy's so fat we won't be able to get him in there with a hundred shoe horns and a bucket of grease!"

The stigma of being obese is terrible. I could have been a drunk or a drug addict, and still be accepted in society because I might be able to hide those things, but being obese, that's impossible to hide and terribly embarrassing. I carried shame everywhere I went.

They brought over the car, and I barely squeezed into it. The salesman asked, "What do you think?"

I said, "Well, I fit," and I just laughed, because I always tried to laugh about things, to kind of ease the situation the best I could. It hurt though, the awkwardness of it all.

The sales guy offered "You wanna go for a test drive?"

I said, "Well, there's no point in going for a test drive. I'll show you a test drive." So I backed it up five feet and I drove it ahead give feet. I said, "It works." What else could I say or do? This was my only choice that would fit, right? I bought that car.

When I first bought it, I would have to move the seat, put it all the way back, put it all the way down to the floor, then put the tilt steering wheel up, make sure it was right up as high as it would go and it would still rub against my belly a bit. I needed a seat belt extension to be able to use the seat belt. Also, I would *always* have to buy a car with a sun roof for the extra headroom and I would still have to bend my neck to keep me from bumping my head off the ceiling.

I used to get pulled over by the cops once in a while, for no seatbelt. I remember this one day a police officer pulled me over and he asked, "You're not wearing a seatbelt, sir?"

I replied, "No."

He asked, "How come?"

I just honestly confessed, "It doesn't fit."

"Oh," he said, "Have a good day." He let me go without a ticket. I was pulled over a few times for various reasons and the cops were always kind when it came to the seatbelt violation, I would just be honest with them and say, "It just doesn't fit." What a dismal way to live. Nothing fit.

The Work Bus — I will share a story later to really unpack the details, but suffice to say I was too big to take the bus. Suncor had these big, beautiful coach buses that came close to my house that would pick up the employees and take us to work, for free. I was too embarrassed to try to squeeze into a single bus seat, so I would just drive into work, that was easily costing me $6000 in extra car expenses every year. The ironic thing is that this embarrassment that I was avoiding for over a decade, never taking the bus, was the same shame that slapped me in the face and woke me up when I was forced to take the bus during that second evacuation.

Shoe Issues — Because I couldn't physically manage to get a pair of socks on, and because I had stinky feet, I'd go through shoes quickly. I handicapped myself by choice, overeating so much and becoming so large that I was no longer able to put on socks. I was also not physically capable of tying laces on shoes. I tried to find those ugly Velcro running shoes. I went to Payless shoes, because they were the only store in town where I used to find these hideous Velcro-strapped laceless shoes. I'd wear them year 'round. They weren't very warm or insulated, but if they had two or three pairs in stock, I would buy them all.

I used to keep a pair that I would leave unworn, virtually brand new, because, sorry, I'm not trying to be gross, but my feet would smell awful without me wearing socks. If I went down south to see Emma in Red Deer, I would take the unworn shoes and wear them because they wouldn't stink as much. If we were travelling we would be in the hotel together, or anywhere that shoes would be taken off and it wouldn't be so bad if I wore my newest pair.

There were many little tricks like that I would need to keep my life as close to "normal" as possible. I'd get baby powder to put it in my velcro shoes to keep the odour at a minimum.

That shoe topic brings another social consequence of obesity into the picture because if your feet stink, you can't go into anybody's home to visit. Here in Canada, it's tradition to take your shoes off when you enter a home. It's a part of Canadian culture. If I would be at a friends house, they would invite me in, but I'd always say, "No. No thanks, I gotta run." I would make up something to avoid entering, to avoid taking off my shoes and doing serious carpet damage. Can you imagine that? Taking my shoes off would have been like a skunk getting loose and spraying everything in sight. No thanks! I would rather just walk out before I had to take my shoes off. That really limited a lot of my social activity.

I would travel to Red Deer to see Emma and even though her mom and I are not dating any longer and haven't been together for over a decade, we have continued to be good friends. As I mentioned, I'm still close with all her family. They are all lovely and welcoming people. The whole family has accepted me. Any time I'd be at any of their homes to drop off Emma or pick her up, they were always inviting me in, but I had to decline the offer for many years because my feet would reek.

With the obesity, my left foot would twist to the outside. The arch would stick up a few inches and I would kind of walk on the side of my foot. After walking that way for months, the sides of my work boots would break and these expensive boots would be wrecked. I could never do my work boots up, the laces were too hard to reach and tie up. I'd take my foot and slide it down into the boot with no sock because I couldn't bend over to tie them up. As a result, my foot would be sliding around in there all day. Work boots on the cement floor with no socks and a loose boot were brutal. By 3:00 o'clock with five hours left to go on my shift, it was like somebody took a sledge hammer right to the bottom of my foot and the left foot was the worst. My feet were a terrible source of pain every day when I was huge.

The Couch — I would look at the couch in my apartment and be disgusted. The couch was dirty, it was sagging, it was broken, reminding me that my couch was like that because I was so incredibly big. I'd go into my bedroom and see the mattress sagging, the banana bed. The couch though, was my daily reminder of what a mess my life was; that's where I spent most of my waking hours. It was also a mess because that's where I did most of my eating and spilling. As the song says "there was always something there to remind me." That was my couch; the only thing I had to sit on.

I didn't really care too much though because nobody really came over anyway. The couch also reminded me that I was alone. Everything reminded me of how big I was and how much my life sucked.

Sore, Stiff, Tingly — Every. Single. Morning.

I never woke up feeling refreshed. It was mental relief to sleep all night and escape reality for a few hours, but there wasn't much physical relief. As I mentioned, I would lose circulation and I would wake up on pins and needles. My muscles were always sore and I always felt stiff and achy all over my body from sleeping on a mattress that was designed to hold people who weigh 300 pounds or less.

Chafing — The chafing on various parts of my body was very painful at times. Underneath my belly, where fat would overhang my belt, it would get raw from friction and perspiration that wouldn't allow my skin to dry properly. Not to sound disgusting, but I would get home from work, I'd lift up my belly and there'd be lots of blood there. I would have to get in the shower and lift up my belly and pour hot water right onto the open chafing. That was horrific pain, but I had to. I found after the hot water, it would kind of feel soothed afterwards. Then I would take Vaseline or baby powder and put it under my belly. After a while, I started taking cloth and I would put it on the inside of my belly, to keep it from chafing. Imagine that! I was incredibly adaptable to learn new ways to survive my obesity, protecting myself, insulating myself so I could continue in this insanity, this lie! Again, I'm not trying to be gross, I just want to give you an accurate picture of how extreme my life was being almost six hundred pounds!

That seemed to help the chafing pain somewhat, but the cloth would cause other things to…I don't know… there's no easy way to say it… it didn't *smell* the best. On hot days, I would get chafing on my legs. As I would walk, I'd have pain in my feet, but then in between my thighs, it was rubbing together. When I got home, in the mirror I would see a lot of redness on the inside of my legs. There's nothing I could do really. I tried buying longer boxers; that kind of helped, but not much. Baby powder helped a bit too.

Restroom — When I was almost 600 pounds even using

the restroom was hard. Life is not designed for people that size. I've already mentioned how my diet was limited at work due to difficulty using washrooms that are too small for the obese population.

I would often look for handicapped stalls in public washrooms to cope. If I went into public restroom and they had a handicapped stall it was like I had it made, "Woo hoo, they have a handicapped stall." As I said, regular sized stalls are not designed for clinically obese people. I was way beyond clinically obese. If I did find handicapped bathrooms I'd make note of it and return to those restaurants or stores.

Having a shower is very difficult, I would barely fit into an average shower stall if I had to shower elsewhere. If I was showering in my own tub I always used to worry, because if I fell down and broke a leg or something I would have been in big trouble.

THE PHYSICAL PARTS are not the full extent of what it means to be clinically obese. There are mental, emotional, social and I suppose even spiritual components to this journey of being such a great weight. Let me try to describe some of these for you:

The Emma Part

I really enjoyed spending time with Emma, especially at the park. I loved doing that. I also loved travelling with Emma. I remember our first little trip together. I think she was seven. Emma and I went down to Drumheller, just for three days. It's the home of Dinosaur Provincial Park, the Royal Tyrrell Museum (one of the premier Dino-Museums in the world) and all kinds of touristy dinosaur attractions. Emma gave me something then. She gave me a little dolphin. It hangs on a little string. To this day, I have that hanging in my car. That represents a precious little token of our first overnight road trip together.

I think she was about seven years old when we took that extended trip. Dinosaurs are magical to almost any seven-year old. I still look over the photos captured during that trip every now and then at home. I look back on those special moments with a big smile on my face. She always had my heart. She's the best thing that ever happened to me.

Emma and I also made a couple of trips to Victoria, B.C.; we drove once and we flew once. I remember when we flew there, that was a bit of an experience because I was huge at the time. Getting on the plane was a painful event. I remember that particular trip vividly. It was me, it was her, and there was another gentleman on the end of the row fitting into three seats. There were only the three of us, but she was feeling crushed between me and the other gentleman because I was so big, taking up a seat and a half. I wasn't even at my biggest then.

I put the armrest up, but I was really crowding into her seat quite a bit. She was just little. Feeling squished, she actually moved to another seat a few rows back and I felt awful because she thought she was making me sad. I looked back a couple times to check on her and saw her sitting there in another row. She had a little frown on her face. I was heart broken to see her sad.

The poor little thing just wanted to be comfortable but she was afraid she had hurt my feelings by moving to a less crowded area. I said, "It's all good, Emma. It's all good," trying to reassure her.

She's always been very protective of me, very sensitive towards me. She would often catch people staring at me and she would glare right back at them. She didn't care how big I was. Ever. She just accepted me. I was her dad and she was proud of me. She was concerned about me. She didn't care about the smell from my feet. She didn't care about me being too big to go out wearing anything but gym pants and a stained t-shirt. She didn't care about any of that. She just accepted me. It was nice. When I spent time with Emma, it was like an escape. There were no judging eyes. There was no pressure. There was nothing negative. It was just her and me.

She has always called me "dad." She still calls me dad. I'm her dad. I'd die for her in a heartbeat if I needed to. It breaks my heart though because a lot of times, as I think back on it, we would do things together and because I was so huge, there were lots of things I could *not* do with her.

I remember one time going to Calaway Park, the big amusement park just west of Calgary, near the Canadian Rockies. I was too big to go on *any* of the rides with her. There was this one ride she desperately wanted to go on. It was Timber Falls, one of their most popular rides. It's a typical amusement park log ride where a final big descent and splash down into a big pool of water is the highlight at the end of the ride. Some of the occupants usually get soaked, the perfect ending on a hot summer day. I went through the long line-up with her, but in the end, just before the ride, she had to get on the Timber Falls ride with another family because I was too big to ride with her. She never complained, not a word. She really wanted to get on that ride *with her dad*, but I could tell she was disappointed. I mean, I could see on her face she was nervous, but she was brave, this little girl, getting into a log with a family of strangers because she really wanted to go on the ride, but she also really wanted to enjoy that ride with her dad — the big guy — too big to fit into a narrow log.

I stood by a fence, near the end of the ride where I could watch the ride come down and make it's big splash. Everything in me wanted to be on that ride with her, to enjoy those magical moments with her and I couldn't because I was too big. I had inadvertently made a choice to spectate rather than participate because I had been selfish by gaining weight. There are too many reminders like that, disappointing memories where I wish I could take the body that I'm in now and go back to her younger years and do all those daddy—daughter moments again because there was so much, so many events and occasions where I missed out.

That's my biggest regret.

My biggest regret is not my health issues or the loneliness. It's the years I have lost, hundreds of moments I missed out on with my daughter because the extra weight I carried took all of that away from me. People ask me, "Why don't you accept treats or have some chocolate, or a donut or ice cream now?" Why would I ever do that? No way! Eating junk food stole that away from me. I hate that junk now. I absolutely hate it. It's like if I was married, and my wife cheated on me. If I met that guy, the guy that took away everything that was dear to me I would not look at him in a positive way. I'd obviously be very upset with him.

That's the way I look at junk food. It took away such a huge part of my life, I'm angry with it. I used to love it, or at least I loved how it made me feel for a few seconds, but now I hate it. I almost look at it like a person. "You came into my life. You stole everything of value from me and you almost killed me. You took away memories. You took away everything I hold dear. I absolutely despise you now and I will never forgive you. I hate you junk food!"

What a rip off! I couldn't even just to go for a walk with Emma because I couldn't walk very far. Visiting a park, I couldn't even get on the swings with her. I couldn't possibly fit into any of those simple little things like a swing in a public park. I could push her on the swing, but I couldn't swing along beside her.

We would go to the mall together. She'd be walking real slow, but she'd be way ahead of me. I'd be lagging far behind. I'd say, "Emma, I've got to sit down for a bit." My feet would be killing me. Everything in my body would be aching. I'd usually be out of breath.

Going to a restaurant with her would be an issue. We would have to make sure that we were seated at a table. I could never fit into a booth. I think most normal-sized people prefer a booth, it's more cozy and quiet. When we would go into the restaurant, I would have to ask first thing, "Can I have a table please?" I just couldn't fit into a booth. Emma would never say anything. She was always very sweet to me, and very protective. She loved me for who I was. She never showed any embarrassment.

My friends were kind and protective as well. I was very fortunate because everybody that I had in my life, the friends and family that I still have in my life, they didn't see the extra 337 pounds on me. They saw my personality, they saw my heart and they looked past all of the surface appearances. They weren't ashamed to be seen with me. I was more ashamed to go out in public than they were to be seen with me.

Emma has her mother's independence. She has her mother's strength. I can be fairly sensitive. She has that tender side of me and she has my sense of humour. Her mother says Emma has my dry sense of humour. Even though she's not technically, biologically mine, she has quite a bit of my personality. She's mine in every sense of the word. The best words I can ever hear are these: "I love you, Dad."

I couldn't continue in life with that amount of weight on my body and expect to live to be an old man. I was already getting the signs of it. Mainly, my legs were tingling, I was getting brown skin on my forehead, my eyes were leaking and I was getting chest pains. I didn't talk about it, but I knew the body was starting to give me signs insisting, "Hey, mister, you better smarten up here. You don't have a lot of time."

I would get a sharp pain every now and then. I wouldn't let Emma know. There were a couple times where I'd get a sharp pain, but I wasn't going to go to the hospital. Not a chance. I don't get those sharp chest pains anymore, not since I lost all the weight. When I was at my heaviest weight the possibility of a heart-attack was always in the back of my mind. It was a thought in Emma's mind too, especially after the panic attack after learning about heart disease in school. How strong is my heart?

When I look back on the situation with Emma now, I think about what a selfish person I was. When my daughter had a panic attack in school, when I was aware of how vulnerable my health was because of my weight, when I couldn't sit beside my little girl at a movie or get a booth in a restaurant or even travel to visit my parents... that was insane. That was nothing but blind selfishness. Even though I was affecting other people, regardless of how much I didn't like myself, I did nothing to change. I had put myself in that condition of being terribly overweight. Obviously, I didn't love myself very much to do that to my own body. But other people still loved me and I was really hurting them, especially Emma.

There's no other word to describe it but selfishness, to eat what I ate, to do that to my body and not care about it, I was being very selfish. I would always think in the back of my mind that I wanted to change and think that I was very vulnerable to all kinds of health conditions, but that still wasn't enough to get me to change.

"Smarten up!" What was I thinking?

There's another vital thing I need to say to anybody who's reading this book. There are people in your life, whether you think it or not, that do love and care about you. Stop being selfish. Change! You're not going to be here forever. None of us are. If you keep doing terrible things to your body, you're really shortening your time. I was slowly killing myself with food. I was robbing Emma every step of the way!

The Being Alone Part

What's it like, being all alone, being that big? I'd say for me, that was a significant negative part of being obese. On a pain scale of 1 - 10, I'd say the pain of being alone was a 7, a very strong feeling.

In the last ten years, I worked eight Christmases. Even if I'm not scheduled to work I will usually take a shift on Christmas day, especially since my daughter moved down to Red Deer. It's good for me to work on Christmas Day. Then I'm not alone, at home, feeling sorry for myself, plus, I get paid holiday and overtime wages. I hate being alone in a lot of ways. Sure I like privacy, I liked how being alone can cover up the shame of habitual over-eating, but the misery of being alone, that's the worst.

Once in a while I might go to a movie alone, but I would only do that on a weekday and I'd go to the late show; I knew hardly anybody'd be there to stare at the fat guy. The seats didn't fit very well. It was an older theatre in Fort McMurray, the kind where I couldn't put the armrest up. I would find a seat next to the main aisle, because they were a little larger, so I'd try to find one of those. I'd try to sit where nobody noticed me.

I didn't really go to church very often because there were crowds. I didn't like being in crowds. I hated going out in public. I enjoy church, but not when it felt like many eyes were on me.

I couldn't go to people's houses because my feet stank. I used to get invited, people would invite me over, but I'd say "No." I'd make up some excuse, but I knew my feet smelled. I knew that if I could smell me, other people could too; not to be disgusting, but those unfortunate realities all came with the territory. I didn't go anywhere. I'd go for a little drive, I'd go get fast food, I'd go to the occasional movie and I'd stay home. The only place I went consistently was work. I'd go down and see my daughter in Red Deer. When I went down to see her we'd just get dinner and a movie, because I hated being in public. I hated being around people who I felt were staring at the big guy. I avoided people, especially crowds of people. I hated being alone, but I preferred to be alone. It was a very awkward and painful time for me.

Anti-Social — I used to be a more social person when I was younger but for fourteen years I felt I was kind of trapped inside that huge body and lost most of my sociable side. That made me feel depressed. In my mind, I knew who I was and I knew how I could be. I saw all my friends going out and I saw all the things I wanted to participate in. I knew I wanted to do things, I wanted to enjoy life, but I couldn't. I had three hundred and fifty extra pounds weighing me down. All of that sucked the life out of me, made me depressed and then I'd just want to eat more. I had nothing to do, I was bored to death. What was there to do? I'd be stuck sitting in my condo, so what could I do?

"Ah, well...I guess I'll go get some more food. All by myself." I had a couple friends that would come over and visit sometimes, but besides that, I wouldn't go anywhere. Like MacAulay Calkin, I'd just be *home alone*.

When I was that size, that was always the worst feeling. Always. Being. Alone.

I'd get up in the morning and on top of everything that I would have to deal with throughout the day, I always felt like nobody else knew what I was dealing with being obese. I felt all alone in the world and I used to dream of having a person that could approach me and say, "You're not alone in this. I've experienced this. I know exactly what you're going through."

I used to wish that I could see somebody, talk to somebody that was going through what I was going through, but had survived and actually changed their life. Most days, that was the hardest part. I guess I was alone physically all the time and I was feeling mentally and emotionally isolated because I didn't think anybody else in the whole world knew what I was going through. I felt nobody could relate to me. I guess the heaviness of that became overwhelming. Not only was I alone physically, but I was alone mentally and emotionally.

I knew what kind of desperation and sadness that brought on me. If I can stress to this to anybody feeling alone, I honestly believe this, if you can get over the feeling that you're not alone in this journey, then you can make it, you can survive, you can move on and you can do something about it. For me, there's no worse feeling than being alone.

I had an upbringing in a home that wasn't perfect by any means, but a home where Christianity was believed and practiced, not just church culture, but real and genuine Christianity. I think, from my reading of the Bible, that when Jesus was on the cross, dying for the sins of the world, He felt absolutely alone. That's God-awful. Jesus was willingly nailed to the cross, nails through his hands or wrists, going through all the pain, having been beaten with fists, whipped and bleeding across his back, wearing a "crown" of thorns pressed into his head and one thing was going through his mind and then came out of his mouth - "My God, my God, why have you forsaken me?"

He was all alone. There's no worse feeling. That feeling applies to every negative situation throughout life. Whatever the "cross", whatever the struggle, the physical pain probably doesn't match the loneliness that I was feeling. It doesn't compare. It's not even close.

The Family Part

I have a friend of mine down East who's been in touch with me a couple times, who wrote me when I was first losing weight and I'll never forget what he said, "It's not only the weight that I've put on, I see what I've done to my kids. We're all big, the whole family." He's struggled a lot with his weight his whole life. The bigger pain for him was how he was hurting his family! Eating poorly had become his family culture.

Since everybody in his family was overweight, it bothered him to realize his kids were over weight. Over-eating had become the norm. In a way, it was easier for the kids to be bigger, because it was the family way, they all understood each other, they appreciated what each other was going through. To have that extra bag of chips, to have the ice cream, to not exercise, not go for walks, that was just normal.

Whether it's a family culture of food abuse or another close community that drags you down, like any addiction, it's important to get away from a negative environment and surround yourself with community or family that can make the lifestyle change with you. United we stand!

The Imprisoned Part

I felt trapped, I felt like I was in prison being 567 pounds. Everybody goes through difficult things, but a lot of people survive difficulty because they have people to help them go through it. A lot of my family lived in Newfoundland. Being so large I was not able to fly home. I needed an extended time to take off work to drive down to the east coast because I was too big to fit on comfortably on a plane. I felt I was trapped in Fort McMurray, thousands of miles away.

There was one stretch that was *seven years* before I got home. Every Christmas, birthday, holidays and every special event I was by myself. Emma, my daughter, she moved down to Red Deer when she was about 10 years old. That was hard. They moved down there, I was still in Fort McMurray six hours away; I felt isolated or trapped geographically. Whether it had been a short distance or long, either way, I felt trapped and far away from family.

I couldn't fly. I couldn't rent a car. Newfoundland takes a weeks drive to get to from Fort McMurray. I remained in a prison in my little town, in my obese little world, unable to travel. Unable to get a booth at the restaurant, unable to walk anywhere, unable to get in another car, a friends or a rental, unable to take my shoes off, unable to shop at a normal store. I felt stuck. I felt like I was in prison.

The Dating Part

Being a big guy I wasn't going to ask a girl on a date. I wasn't exactly in the place where I could be "picking up chicks". At almost 600 pounds, the last place I wanted to be was in a crowd of people, let alone attempting to approach an attractive woman and ask, "Hey, would you want to go out on a date with me," while wearing my best pair of stained gym pants and my best t-shirt with only a couple stains on it. I didn't have the confidence to approach people, especially pretty ones.

It's already scary enough to be out in public, it's even worse to imagine asking a lady to go out on a date. It's hard enough to ask a woman out when you're a half decent man, not to mention a man of the 600-pound-variety. I was just always alone.

In a normal world, social activities that would make a person happy, like going bowling with friends, or going to a movie, or grabbing a coffee or even running some errands — normally a person would feel some connectedness doing those things with other people. We might feel a sense of community, a sense of belonging. To go on a date, a person could feel a wonderful sense of companionship or acceptance. To have a person ask you out or to accept a date with you — that feels terrific! To be admired or to have your admiration returned with a, "Sure, I'll go out with you", even if it's just one date, that feels pretty special. I didn't have any of that. I had a couple friends that would drop by and visit and hang out on my banana couch. That was nice. We'd meet for a coffee. Outside of that, there was nothing. I was just always by myself.

The Spare Time Part

My leisure activity was food. I'd order wings and I'd order a lot of different take out foods. I'd go to KFC and get a 10 piece bucket for myself. That was my hobby. For that brief moment when I would get that junk food, or I would get that takeout, for that brief moment, I had happiness. That was what I did in my spare time, my hobby. It was all in that bucket of chicken or whatever I was eating. There were no problems, there was nothing to bother me. I felt good for a few seconds because I had sweet, greasy, salty or some form of happy food in that moment. I would feel joy for a minute, and then I would feel misery for hours.

Loss of Intimacy

I did an interview one time on a radio show in Edmonton, the Pepper & Dylan Show — comedians. One of them asked, "So, what was your sex life like when you were that size?"

I said, "Well, picture two pillows trying to go at it."

He started laughing. He said, "What?"

I said, "There is no sex life, what are you talking about? My sex life was a bag of chips. That was the only love in my life." He just laughed, but it's really sad.

There's another thing to consider when we talk about intimacy, I mean, the physical intimacy. A woman wants to be loved and cherished. For a man, it's sometimes just about the physical attraction, but a woman wants the emotional intimacy, the connection, the tenderness and the care. In my opinion for a woman it's a lot harder to be overweight than a man. I suppose it's a compliment to women, because ladies will look beyond a man's appearance and look to their heart for intimacy.

Men can be a lot like savage dogs. I think the first thing most men consider is a woman's appearance. Women know that. I think it's very hard for a woman's self-esteem if they carry extra weight, a lot more difficult, I think, than it is for men. I feel for overweight women more than men, to be honest. I really do. I'm sorry, but we men can really be insensitive, shallow jerks, not seeing the value of deeper emotional connection.

Being almost 600 pounds, I didn't see any emotional or physical connection. I only picked up on the vibe of disdain, repulsive feelings of rejection. There was no intimacy of any sort being obese.

The Angry Part

When I was a huge size, 6XL and 7XL, with a 66-inch waist that was too tight, the littlest things would really get to me. *Every* little thing would tick me off or make me very angry. I was frequently frustrated and irritated. I would easily fly off the handle when the slightest thing didn't go my way. I remember one morning I got up to go to work and I felt I couldn't go to work unless I had a Diet Pepsi. There was rarely a time that my cupboard was bare in terms of Diet Pepsi on hand. It was my energy and caffeine pipeline. This one particular morning I thought I still had some at home, but for some reason I never reloaded the supply the night before.

I went to work and I was determined that I was going to get some of my beloved "black gold" out of the vending machine and I inserted a $20 bill. That lousy machine took my $20 bill and only gave me one Diet Pepsi, no change. Unbelievable! That really ticked me off. That set me right off the deep end. I went over to the tire shop where I work and we'll just say the boys *knew* I was in a bad mood.

That's the most expensive Diet Pepsi I've ever had.

One of the guys at the shop, left and came back shortly after and rescued me with soda. I'm not sure where he found some product. I don't know if they got the machine working, if he robbed a Pepsi truck, or what he did. I really didn't care. He managed to get me a couple of those life-saving Diet Pepsis and a bag of hickory sticks.

It was those kind of little things going wrong that would get to me. I realize now that when I was in pain, constantly, chronically, day-to-day, every day, dealing with all kinds of emotional tension, all the complications from being that size, the loneliness, the family issues, the loss of freedom, everything involved with being obese, then those little things would get to me and I would realize how angry and frustrated I really was. I was miserable. I was imprisoned in a 600-pound frame. I was there by my own foolish and selfish choices. I hated myself for it.

It was a living hell being obese.

6

The Winds of Change

Growing up in the Northern Peninsula of Newfoundland facing the great Atlantic Ocean was an amazing privilege. I've seen some of the fiercest storms, harshest temperatures and strongest winds that many people will never see. Having the pleasure of growing up on a boat and having a fisherman as my father, I learned a thing or two about the skies, the sea and the wind.

If a heavy storm was brewing over Greenland and a Nor'Easter was heading our way, Dad knew it long before the weather reports did. If a warmer front was heading up the Gulf Stream from the south, it affected the cod long before a promise of warmer days was in the newspaper. When those subtle or major changes were coming up the coast, the fishermen had their ways of knowing the winds of change were on their way. Something was about to shift and we were ready for it.

This story is based around the wildfires in Fort McMurray, but I was ready for a change before that. I was sick and tired of being sick and tired. My life wasn't happy for years leading up to the fire. In my heart and in my mind I was ready for the winds of change. I was ready for a jolt back to reality and the fires of 2016 brought exactly that.

They say the definition of insanity is "doing the same thing over and over again and expecting different results." That's the first half of my story in a nutshell. To be honest, I knew I was going no where fast. I had tried dieting many times, made dozens of excuses over and over, fell short literally over a hundred times and I knew I needed to change.

Those eye-opening "events" on the bus and the plane made it obvious. My life wasn't working. My life was not working. My lifestyle wasn't working. I wasn't happy. I don't know what I was waiting for - death maybe? I don't even know. What I *do* know is my attitude needed to change much more than it had before; I needed a BIG change. As the old saying goes, "desperate times call for desperate measures."

More than Surviving

As an obese person, day-to-day survival got me used to living on my own and doing things myself. I became very stubborn and very independent. Not only was I dealing with shame and embarrassment, but I also had to deal with constant physical pain, mental torment and loneliness. Loneliness, not just from living in isolated north east Fort McMurray, Alberta, but living alone, forty-three and not married and never been married. Emma lives far away from me and my family is in Newfoundland. I have work friends, but outside of that, there's just me, alone, being stubborn and independent.

I think that's a big factor in why I lost the weight. As I became more and more stubborn I learned that dieting, well, actually changing my whole lifestyle with eating and walking was just another thing that I had to do, there was no choice. No one else was going to take charge of my life and fix it, so I had to suck it up and just do it. That strong independence, that stubbornness has been an advantage of being that size; being huge taught me how to get thin again. Those difficulties built character, a mental strength and perseverance found only in the tough times.

I finally realized, if I'm not going to change my life by myself, nobody is going to do it for me. I still have to go to work, I still have bills to pay. I have to clean my house and take out the garbage. Life goes on every single day. I felt I had to have the attitude to suck it up and get 'er done. I needed to ignore everything else and learn quite a bit of stubbornness, resilience and independence.

There's no limit to the possibilities once you have faced the impossible and overcome it. I haven't had any processed sugar in two and a half years. None.

I would always hear an inner voice when I was overweight. It was always there in my head from the time I woke up in the morning until I went to bed at night. I was constantly knowing that I had to become somebody else, somebody different. I couldn't keep going on like this. I was constantly wishing that I could be *somebody else*. I would buy junk food but something in my head was saying, "this has to stop."

To silence that voice, I would continually lie to myself. I'd always make myself fake promises and convince myself with all kinds of lies. Once I had convinced myself of these lies, it made it easier to go buy the junk food. Essentially, I was saying, "This is only temporary. There is an end to this misery coming. I'm going to have a whole new life soon, down the road. I'll enjoy these last couple of days." I was constantly enabling myself. That's how I got through years of obesity.

When that time would come to start the diet, to keep my word to myself, I'd keep lying, telling myself, "I'm going to start my diet today." It might literally only last one hour. I'd go to the grocery store to start buying healthy food and I'd see my favourite junk foods and convince myself, "That looks good. It's on sale. They've got my favourite ice cream right there." I'd even look on the bag of chips and see the expiry date was far down the road. "Wow, now I know these are super fresh. It's almost like I'm buying fresh vegetables. What's another week? I'll start eating healthy next week. Oh, it's too close to Christmas. I can't diet now, it's too close to my birthday." I made up whatever excuse I could, but really, I was constantly lying to myself.

I kept trying to convince myself, "I've got lots of time," but I knew better; I knew I didn't.

My skin was turning brown. I had dark circles under my eyes. I could hardly get a good nights sleep. I was always exhausted and out of breath.

Seeing those two seats on that bus I knew I was going to have to take both seats. Then, seeing the same problem on the airplane, I knew I wasn't just lying to myself anymore — now I was hurting others. I could lie to myself, but I'm not someone who could lie to or hurt *other* people. Somehow, that lying was unacceptable. Somehow, something finally clicked. I finally said, "this is enough!"

My mind kept rehashing, "What if we got evacuated from that camp that night and a person couldn't sit next to me. What if the next day there was news that one person who wasn't able to be evacuated got killed at that camp?" How could I ever have lived with that? I couldn't. Thank God that didn't happen.

Even beyond the possibility of what could have gone horribly wrong, I had to face what did go wrong. I think about all the worry that taking those extra seats did cause somebody, somewhere. I brought on additional anxiety during the evacuation because I was so large. There was a man's wife, a wife's husband, a parent, a daughter or a son who couldn't get a seat on that plane and had to wait hours for the next plane. Somebody was waiting for them to show up in Edmonton and had to wait longer for their loved ones to get home because I was too overweight.

I was realizing that my weight was having a horrible effect on more people than just myself. I finally had to make a decision to stop being selfish. So what? Lots of people might live selfishly — so what? Why does that matter to me so much? I know I'm still selfish in some ways, but when it comes to my weight I realized I was affecting people's day-to-day lives. Where would it stop? Would I become some sociopath who just kept damaging others and not caring at all?

I guess I knew it was hurting people all along; that bothered me. I cared, but I didn't think it was hurting people that much — I minimized it. I told myself it was no big deal. I lived like an ostrich; I had my head in the sand. Because I have lived alone, and I had no immediate family in Fort McMurray, I could escape the reality of what it was doing to other people. They weren't there, close by every day to remind me. It was not *in my face*.

When guys from work would care about me and say something, if they got in my face a little bit, how could I just "blow it off?" I couldn't blow Corey off. He was forty-three when he died; too young to die. I know Corey was saying things to me, confronting me in love. He cared about me. Corey was one of the strongest people I've ever met. I think about Corey every day, to this day. How could I "blow that off?"

I was walking around near 600 pounds, still in my own little junk food bubble hiding from reality, I could ignore the truth of my problems and stay in denial.

―

FOR SOME REASON, with that fire and with the evacuation, the extra seat I took, that was enough. With everything that went on the day of the evacuation and everything that led up to it, I was finally ready. That was the culmination of all my issues, and I finally said, "This is it. That's enough!"

I REMEMBER, as clear as crystal, being in the plane, looking out the window and seeing the clouds and looking down and seeing all the smoke coming up from the trees and huge columns of smoke filling the sky thinking, "This is it. That's enough!" I don't know if it was the stress of everything, being evacuated for the second time, or just escaping with my life for the second time in as many weeks. Who would hire a 600-pound man if I didn't have a job to go back to, if the fire destroyed everything, if none of us were ever allowed back to Fort McMurray, if it had caused all the oil companies to be shut down and my security and livelihood were taken away?

I started to realize that not only was I affecting other people from being evacuated, but I've also put myself in dire straights. I've painted myself into a corner. I was operating on the minimum, only surviving day-to-day life, just barely getting by. I needed to be honest with myself and make some serious changes.

When something drastic like the evacuation happened, I really wasn't prepared to start over. I don't think I could have done ANY other job. I couldn't even do general labour work. I couldn't fit into a truck. I couldn't drive a pick-up truck. I couldn't fit behind the wheel of a forklift. I couldn't even step on a scale for my annual physical. I could run my machine at work, but that's about all I could do.

Every morning I'd get up, I'd wish I was somebody else. I knew something had to change. I knew something had to be done, but I could never find it in myself to do it — until I had that moment and admitted, "That's enough!"

Handicapped — I handicapped myself. It's like I was in a wheelchair for ten years and then I learned to walk again, but I had been in the wheelchair by choice. I consciously sat down in the wheelchair. I cut off my own legs; that's exactly what I did eating junk for all those years. It sounds absurd, but until I said, "That's enough!" it was like I was okay with that for fourteen years of wasteful life.

I am ashamed of myself because of the disservice I have done to the handicapped community. What they're going through is no fault of their own. They were born with it or circumstances brought about their handicap - a car accident or some other tragedy. I put myself in that same boat voluntarily. I felt very ashamed because there are people that would give anything to be out of that handicapped life and I did it to myself voluntarily for many years.

Attitude is Everything

I'm not sure how I managed to stay as positive as I did considering my state. I suppose a part of it had to do with growing up in a home where the basics of Christianity were truly understood as it applies to character: humility, teachability, being thankful - those kind of things made a huge impact on who I've always been, or at least who I've tried to be.

I felt I had to stay positive. I feel that if you have given up being positive, it's like you're already dead inside. Not the fake kind of positive that continually says, "I'm doing great," with a phoney smile. For me, real life had to keep rolling along. I still had to get up in the morning and go to work. I still had to interact with people. I still had a daughter I had to look after. I still had a mortgage to pay. I still have my family back east that I try to be in touch with and help when I can.

With all of that going on, either I get up in the morning, or I quit and die. I've made a choice to keep going. Every day starts and I have another day in front of me; the sun keeps rising and setting. Nothing is going to change physically with me, whether I'm angry or not, sad or happy. Who doesn't wish they were happy? If I go around all day being that extra large size, mad at the world all the time, then I'm going to end up being very lonely.

There were days I went to work, and I was just in a bad mood. Everybody has bad days, but when you're that size, I guess I had a few more. For the most part I was a generally happy guy. I just had to find it in me. I just had to suck it up and do my job well because others were counting on me. I had to find some things to be happy about; little things to look forward to, any positive thing really but to me it was almost always food.

I had to believe that it was possible to be positive in any situation. I could make my environment better if I looked on the bright side. We are not just thermometers, we are thermostats. We don't just read the situation, we help create the environment. I always go back to this same thought, *I have got to make my own happiness.* There's nobody responsible for my life but me. If I'm in a toxic environment, or if I have negative friends pulling me down, there's no excuse, I have to take responsibility for myself and get out of that negative situation.

We only get one shot at this. Ultimately, I'm the only one that's going to do anything about my own situation. If my friends, or even family for that matter, if they're causing me to be stressed, if I can't help but be toxic when I'm around them, drinking, abusing drugs, overeating or whatever I'm doing out of bounds, then I have to remove myself from that. I have to make changes.

There are no real excuses. There are no valid excuses.

Changing My Stinking Thinking

My thinking was messed up. That's what needed to change. I was thinking, when I was at my lowest, it's almost like the message in my head was, to me personally, "Tony, you're completely alone. Nobody really gives a crap about you (although people did), you're completely alone, so who cares? Just abuse your body and eat whatever food you want. It's all that's going to make you happy."

Now the message I get, since I've lost the weight, is "Tony, ultimately you're by yourself and you're responsible for your own decisions. You've only got one life to live. Ultimately, it's your responsibility that you got this obese. You did it alone and it's only you that's going to make the changes to get this weight off." That's how I think now, with a big focus on self-responsibility; it was me and only me that put that weight on. It's only me that can reverse the trend.

All these people that have been very successful in their lives, they've never given up. They've been through failure, after failure, after failure. I'm sure Bill Gates tried all kinds of things that didn't work. Thomas Edison obviously learned from his many failed attempts, Albert Einstein made mistakes, I'm sure. All these amazing men, they were all "failures" at different points in time. It's the same with weight loss.

If there's one thing I would like to get through to people, it's the message, "Don't give up!" We only truly fail if we stop trying. Eventually something will stick. Eventually something will come into our lives, into our thinking and we'll discover, that there are things much more important than making ourselves feel good through food by "treating" ourselves. We'll find something that will click somehow, we will find other things in life that we can use as a treat. There are other things in life to make us happy besides food.

It's all about the mind. It's the mind that makes people

depressed, it's the mind that convinces people that they're useless or that they don't even want to wake up in the morning. It's also the mind that can get me out of bed at 5:00 in the morning at minus 40, to go for a walk, because I realize that my body is worth it.

If your mind is telling you, "I need you to walk two kilometres a day, to get in shape because I need you not to die." Somehow we can ignore that. Don't we care enough about ourselves to listen to our bodies screaming for attention and help? My point is this: **if we could only love ourselves as much as we love our family we would be a lot better off. It would be great if we could do as much for ourselves as we do for our family.** Why don't we? It's like that analogy of being on a plane. The flight attendants remind us before taking off that if the oxygen mask drops down, we need to put the oxygen mask on our own faces first, before we help our neighbour. That's the way it should be with weight loss: I valued everybody else around me, friends and family, but I didn't value myself, yet I'm no good to everybody else if I'm no good to myself. It means taking a lot of self-responsibility. If we can unlock that potential in our mind, then we can do whatever we want and help whoever we want to help.

You can fix this. If I can fix what's going on in my head, then I can do anything. If there's anything I've learned through all this and I'm not trying to sound cliché, but the main thing that's really stopping us from reaching our goals, it's our own thinking. If we'll just realize that there's nothing that can stop us once we get our heads sorted, we can do whatever we set our minds to do. I was 41 years old. I was almost 600 pounds. I didn't join a gym. I didn't go on any special diet, I just lost the weight "naturally". The only thing that changed in all of that, and in my whole life was that something changed in my head. ***I changed my stinkin' thinkin'!***

That's what happened when I saw the extra seat I was

stealing from somebody else on the evacuation bus and on the airplane. My thinking changed. Enough was enough. That switch went off!

We need to change and engage our minds immediately because time keeps moving on. It's going to keep moving regardless of what we do. Regardless of what kind of life we choose to live, the clock is ticking. I lost 337 pounds in about two years. Two years is nothing! It's twenty-four months. That goes by in a blink of an eye. I just needed to wake up and realize I was almost 600 pounds! I needed to face the fact that a normal chair could barely hold my weight - or maybe not. At any time I could have just been honest with myself and convinced myself, "Twenty-four months is all it will take if I eat clean, no sugar and limit my carbs. In twenty-four months I can have a wonderful life, or if I don't do anything, in twenty-four months I could possibly be dead."

Time can be your friend, or it can be your enemy. Two years is not much time, compared to your whole life. It's going be hard, I'm not going to lie, it will take a lot of sacrifice to get the life you really want. The possibility for transformation is limitless when a person can look at their situation and say, "Sure it's going to be hard, but it's only a short season to sacrifice to get there, then I have my entire life ahead of me and I can live with a much better quality of life."

If I don't pay that price a year or two years goes by and I'm still stuck in a bad situation. Add another two years and another two years… Next thing I know, ten years has gone by and I'll never get that time back again. I'm still going to have to make that hard decision to change, or die the same - probably a lot sooner. Why wait?

I was sitting down with a friend. He's an alcoholic and drug addict. He's dealing with some major stuff, but he's a wonderful guy at heart. I looked at him and said, "You know what? You will quit drinking. You will quit drugs." He looked a little surprised and he said, "How do you know that Tony?"

I said, "You'll either do it by force, or you're going to do it voluntarily, but eventually, you will stop. You might be six feet under, but you will stop. It's up to you to choose how you're going to do it." It's choices. It's all in our thinking, in our thought processes, in my opinion, thinking is the game-changer. If we can win the battle inside our heads, we're more than half the way there.

I look back and I think only two and a half years ago, it seems like a lifetime ago, but only two and a half years ago, I was that huge, obese man. It seems like a dream come true to lose all this weight. Here I am now enjoying all these experiences. Last week I was in Mexico on vacation. Three years ago I could not physically fit onto a plane. Yesterday I went to my first ever NHL game in Buffalo. I could not physically fit in those kind of arena seats a few years ago; I would have had to get special handicapped seats. All these neat things, two and a half years ago, I never would have thought possible. In the fall of 2015, if you would have told me I would be writing a book about weight loss, I would have said, "I'll make that bet with you right now! Easy money. That's NOT possible!" Right? Yet, here I am writing this book. Once you set your mind to it, you can accomplish so much in such a short amount of time - then you can have the rest of your life to enjoy it.

People may keep on rolling with whatever they're struggling with for years and years and years, thinking they can never get out of it. Whether it's drugs, or alcohol, or a bad marriage, or weight gain, or debt, or anything, time can be your friend. Even if you're struggling financially you can change your thinking. You can decide you want to put away $50 each payday for two years, $100 a month. In two years, you have $2,400 put away. All of a sudden, you have a small little nest egg in your bank account; it's earning interest without even raising a finger, with you doing *nothing*, your money is earning money for you. Any situation can be resolved, if you just make time your friend.

Looking back, I've thought many times, especially when I'm by myself, "This is all just a dream. I still feel like I'm going to wake up and find this was all just a dream."

A friend asked me if I could write a letter, or send a text message to my younger self, in my early twenties knowing what I know now, what would I say to a younger Tony?

I would say, "Take a knife and cut off your finger. That pain will be much less than what you're going to put up with for the next twenty years if you keep going down that path." (Please don't try this at home!) That's what *I* would say *to myself*. I wish I could have come to my senses sooner! I know it's stupid. The pain I've put myself through; emotionally, physically, mentally, financially, socially and romantically. I've hurt myself every way imaginable. Truthfully, losing a finger would have been much less painful. I would add, speaking to my younger self, "Do it while you still have time. Don't waste your life."

I wish I had done it sooner, before I knew Emma or her mom, Penny. How different life might have been. I don't know poetry, but I've heard this short poem that's really impacting:

> "Of all sad words of tongue or pen,
> The saddest are these, "What might have been."

Nobody knows the pain I've been through and the regrets that have come with it. Although I tried to describe it, I can't ever put fully into words the physical and emotional pain that being obese causes. I can't explain fully what it's like.

It's as though you pick up six, or seven water jugs and throw them on your back and walk around with them for ten years. Who would? What area of your life goes unhurt through that? Try putting that on your back and going to work every day! Drive your kids to school with the equivalent of two washing machines in the driver's seat with you. Try going on a date with that baggage on your back. Do your day-to-day errands, drop by the bank, pop into the grocery store, head to the post office. Try to function as a *normal* human being, try doing all that stuff and you still must try to put a smile on your face!?! Good luck with that! Who does that? Who would be dumb enough to carry seven water jugs on their back? I was. Or even one jug? Or even half of a jug? That must even do some damage to your life.

I look back on it now and I don't know how I survived. I have friends that asked me, "I don't know, how did you do it?" I think it's a miracle. This is where the prayers of my mother came into play because there's no other way I naturally could have survived. It doesn't matter what my relationship with God was or is or how much I go to church or didn't. Over the past few years, Mom's prayers worked. God has still been right there helping me out. I know He is there for us all, regardless of what shape we are in. God is still God. He's still up there. Don't mistake His patience or His silence for indifference. I still believe to this day that it was a miracle I survived everything I've been through.

There's no way you can come out of a decade and a half of being that size, carrying all that weight, working full-time, continuing to abuse junk food and still come out with no diabetes, no major problems, nothing wrong. My feet still work. My eyes and skin have recovered. My legs still work. Everything still works. Everything works wonderfully. (But the guys at work might say I'm a little brain damaged). I really do believe it's a miracle I survived.

What if I had been injured while I was almost 600 pounds? It is strange, because when I started losing a lot of weight I *did* get hurt. I was in a few ambulance rides. I had my first problem when I was approximately 160 - 170 pounds lighter. I fell off a stand at work. I was lifting up a piece of steel that normally would have been very easy for me to lift when I was heavy. Your mind still thinks you're 600 pounds, but your body's saying, "You can't lift what you used to be able to lift." I lifted it up and it swung back and hit me. I went down hard. It came down and landed on me. I banged my head hard on the cement floor. At the hospital I was smiling the whole time I was getting stitched up! I wouldn't have fit in an ambulance before, but I could at 400 pounds.

At work, they did an investigation into the accident. My manager told me one of their conclusions, "We basically figured that because you're not used to having your lower weight, your body miscalculated, it's just a lot of adjustments. Years ago, you would have lifted that no problem." I agreed, "Yeah, it wouldn't have been an issue."

One thing I don't have like I used to is strength. It used to be that I could lift or move anything. I could care less about that anymore. With all this weight loss, it has made me strong *mentally*. If I could get through all of that and come out alive, I can do anything. I'm not perfect by any means. I still make plenty of mistakes, but I can — *you can* — deal with anything.

Nothing seems like a problem anymore. To go through that terrible life I had for fourteen years, there's nothing that can get me down now. My thirties were wasted, thrashing in the throes of throbbing loneliness. My forties are going to be phenomenal. My fifties are going to be fabulous. My sixties are going to be sensational. I'm not going to waste time regretting my thirties. I'll just chalk it up to a HUGE learning experience.

If this book is helpful to a few folks, then at least I can say that's one positive thing that came of all that weight gain. I want to get a good message out there and hopefully help people realize their potential. If one person would come up to me or send an email and say, "I read that book and it helped me, it helped to change my life" it would all be worthwhile.

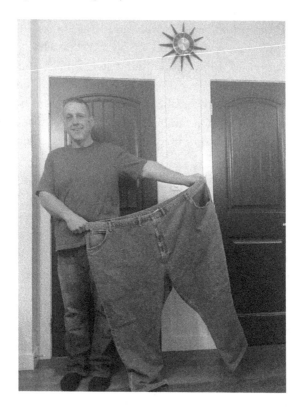

Many of the poor lifestyle or individual life decisions we make are like a bit of temporary insanity. If we balanced the short-term pleasure with the long-term damage, no one in their right mind would make those terrible choices, but that's the issue. I wasn't in my right mind. I was in a short-term selfish insanity that was so extreme it was literally killing me.

I'm not trying to be preachy here, but with a Christian and church background, I can't help but remember that old story of Adam and Eve in the garden of Eden and how the snake tempted them with the forbidden fruit (which the bible never says was an apple by the way — apples are from God, not Satan). I love this about the bible that there are all these little nuggets and details in the stories that offer very useful life lessons. If there is a detail in a bible story that seems obscure there's usually some truth to be found there.

The one detail that kind of cracks me up in the Adam and Eve narrative is the comment the snake makes when he points them to the forbidden fruit (probably potatoes, probably right beside a deep fryer). The snake says, "You will certainly not die!" Wow. That's the first example of a ridiculously exaggerated lie in all of history. That, my friends, is temporary insanity. "Take it, have a little, you'll be fine. Know one will know. You're not hurting anyone else. Go ahead, you're consenting adults. Feel free. Who Cares?" Those little bits of temporary insanity are some of the most damaging, destructive, deadly lies I ever got sucked into - for fourteen years to be precise. That is the subtle deception that almost killed me; temporary insanity.

I had to say "no" to the ice cream and the donuts those early days in Edmonton and Red Deer, for me, I had to be all-in, totally committed to a new way of life. No more treats. No more cheats. No days off. No flexibility. It was so real to me that it really felt like this was my last chance to change. If I don't do it now I'll never do it. What if I don't do it? What would happen?

Eventually I would die. Maybe not this week, not this month, maybe not even this decade but I was choosing a premature death. Could I have had one or two Timbits in Edmonton that first night of evacuation and been fine? Technically, yes, I would have been fine, but realistically and truthfully, no, I would have stayed in the temporary insanity thinking. For me, the open door to selfishness was deadly.

I like the story of the company that was looking for a driver and tested the candidates on their driving skills on a narrow road by a cliff. One driver boasted that he could safely drive within feet of the edge. Another said he could drive safely within inches of the cliff. The third driver asked why anyone in their right mind would drive anywhere near the edge. She would want to stay as far away from the edge as possible. She got the job. Good story! I don't want to be the guy living so close to the edge any more.

If living with clear, strong boundaries and guidelines sounds boring to you, you might be right, but in my case, I'd rather be boring than dead. The thing is, I eat great! I have all kinds of delicious meals and I thoroughly enjoy food. I just don't do so in the temporarily insane way that was killing me. Is there a place of balance in this? Not for me there wasn't. I had to go all—in. I had to sacrifice sugar and all the deep-fried junk food to save my life. I have no regrets.

Three years ago, at that size, I was shortening my life in a huge way. Frequently, I'd go to bed really not knowing if I would wake up. That thought would occur quite often as I was going to bed at night, getting ready, brushing my teeth, taking off my clothes and saying a little prayer, "Lord, forgive me if I've wronged or hurt anyone today. Please forgive my sins. If I don't make it through the night, I need to make my peace with You." That's a very profound thing. That was reality for me.

Please don't think I have this crippling fear of death. I don't. It's quite the opposite really. I don't want to die, and I don't want to die while I'm still pretty young but I'm at peace with it if I do die. One of the blessings of the Christian faith is this sweet assurance I have that if I die I don't have to face eternity alone or with any measure of uncertainty. I have a promise of heaven in the afterlife and a wonderful peace and joy here on earth, right now, every day of this life.

There were times where I would wake up in the mornings surprised I woke up. It was very real to me, because with the condition my body was in, it felt like this was my last chance.

What really helped me with the cravings, in the beginning especially, was this line of thinking in my mind, "I'm doing well. I'm losing weight. If I give in and I have a treat, I'm going to feel horrible for having that treat. I'm going to lose some of the momentum and some of the progress that I've made for a VERY small amount of short-lived pleasure." That short-term pleasure was what had been destroying me for my entire life.

I like that quote attributed to Kate Moss, "Nothing tastes as good as skinny feels." It doesn't even have to be "skinny." In my case, nothing tastes as good as "normal" feels; wearing normal clothes, sitting in a normal seat, lying on a normal mattress. There's a lot of truth to that and I think it reflects the short-term vs. long-term battle with food. Usually we get sucked in to the taste, the flavour, the sugar rush and get stung with the long-term side effects, or we just ignore the reality of the consequences or minimize the consequences all together. If we can get past the short-term pleasure fix that's so huge in our instant-fix-world, we can choose to live in such a way as to achieve our long-term goals.

For me, with food, it was always a very small amount of pleasure that I would escape to, but the reality was still there. It tasted good. I felt nice. I would have that bit of pleasure, but I couldn't escape my reality. It's very hard to put into words, but my thinking was, "I'm hungry. I really feel like my favourite burger. I've been doing great on this diet, I could go have a burger."

However, if I'm honest with myself, I know how I am. I'm really onto my sneaky ways and what I WILL actually do, so the conversation in my head about having a burger continues like this: "Yes, but if I do it once, then I'll do it again. I'm going to do it again. I always do. If I eat that burger, I'm going to feel horrible about eating it because I've been doing so well. And I'd risk putting weight back on if start down that path again, that's a mistake I better not make.

That would be really dumb. If I do have the burger, I'm still going to be hungry within an hour. So, all I will have accomplished, is to make myself feel bad, ruined my diet a little bit and I'll have put myself at risk of gaining weight again for five or ten minutes of pleasure, eating that burger. I better not."

WAS EATING junk ever worth it? When my brain clicked years ago, one thing that I realized was that 10 or 15 minutes of shallow happiness or pleasure just wasn't worth it anymore for me. The guilt, the sadness, the discomfort, the medical issues, the pain and everything that it brought with it; definitely NOT worth it. When I finally clued into that, it made it much easier to not have any junk at all anymore. When I finally clued into the fact that 10 or 15 minutes of a tiny little bit of pleasure was not worth the guilt and all the other countless side-effects. I could finally walk away from that dysfunctional lifestyle. I realized that it's truly easier to give it all up. There's no better satisfaction than eating clean all day. There's no guilt with doing my walks. I could watch my food intake. I could eat healthy and feel awesome.

I'D GET up in the morning and think, "I made it through yesterday!" I'd feel great. I'd feel totally satisfied. I would feel very happy, very pleased with myself. I originally put together a string of three weeks, doing that over, and over, and over, and then I hit the scale at work and realized I'd lost thirty pounds. That was awesome. I continued the string of more days and my belt started getting a bit looser, and my jeans were getting a little looser, I was really making progress. Then more days of consistent stubborn saying "no!" to burgers, junk food, fried chicken; the momentum kept building.

New Attitude

These days I'm much more optimistic than I used to be. I'm wanting to give back, wanting to spend more time with the people I love. I'm more aware of how fragile life is. I'm more appreciative of the limits of time that we have. I'm not as selfish when it comes to how I treat my body, because whether we want to realize it or not, our actions affect those that we love greatly. Putting them through that pain, that's why I feel that I was a selfish idiot. To put them through the pain and the worry of wondering what was going to happen to me was cruel. I was limited in how much time I could spend with the ones I love because of my size. I choose the short-term enjoyment of food over them. That was selfish. That was inconsiderate. They might look at it differently, but I think that I was being incredibly selfish.

Now I'm greatly aware that life is very, very fragile, and we should be doing everything we can to make it last as long as we can and not speed up the process because of our short-sighted choices.

I remember the story of Moses, the great father of the Jewish Faith and leader of the Hebrew people. There's an interesting thought about him in the New Testament scriptures (from the perspective of Christianity looking back on Jewish heroes). It tells us (in Hebrews 11:25) that Moses, who was brought up in a palace as Pharaoh's son, who lived in luxury his whole life, made a choice to be mistreated along with the enslaved Jews, rather than enjoying short-term pleasure. That really challenges me because that is exactly what I did for fourteen years; I chose the short-term joys of sugar and junk food that were slowly killing me. I didn't choose to sacrifice like

Moses did to reach a long-term goal. I only saw the short term. No wonder Moses is considered a hero to Jews and Christians alike.

I'm very aware of how limited time is, through everything I've been through. I'm aware from my friend Corey passing away and seeing others get sick. We can be here today, enjoying life, and a couple days from now any one of us could be involved in a car accident or have some serious medical issue and, boom! Just like that, we're gone. There's no guarantee of tomorrow. There is a lot of responsibility in how we take care of ourselves. The way I took care of myself in my thirties was very selfish, very lazy. I took no pride in who I was, with little or no self care.

It has affected the people that I love terribly. It affected my daughter in that I lost a lot of opportunities to spend quality time with her in some of the best stages of her life. I will never get that back. I lost time in having a relationship with a girlfriend or possibly a wife, or even being able to go out on a date. That is time that I'll never get back. I lost the opportunity of spending time with my parents because I couldn't travel home very often, so they didn't get to see me. That was incredibly selfish on my part. I lost years because of my selfishness, and because of my lack of self worth, of having no pride in my body or giving up and not caring.

I realize it affected many other people. I know that as part of the twelve-step process for recovering addicts, from alcohol or drugs, that step number eight is to make a list of all the people you have hurt and that you need to be willing to make amends to all of them. I'm becoming very aware now just how many people I've hurt with my food addiction.

I can never get that back. I can make money again where I've lost it, but I can't make back or take back time. The only thing I can do that gives me hope is say, "From now on..." I hope and pray to God that I have thirty, forty or fifty years left so that now I can make up for it, but there are no guarantees. I look back on it, especially all the time away from my family back in Newfoundland and all the time I spent away from my daughter down in Red Deer. I look at all the trips I could have made by plane if I was a normal size. I think about all the times that Emma and I could have gone to Calaway Park, a water park, or went on trips together if I was normal size. It's terrible.

I also feel bad about all I put her through with worry, things that I'm sure she never said to me, but I could see by the look on her face that she was worried about me. That's a lot to put a little person through. If I would have had a heart attack and died, that would have just devastated Emma. I am thankful that I finally changed. I'm forty-three and hopefully, I still have quite a few years left in me. I was forty-one and six hundred pounds. If I had never done anything to lose weight, by this age I'm at now, there's a good chance I'd be six feet under.

I clearly remember what my mother said to me one time, after I lost the weight, I'll never forget it. Almost in tears, she told me she used to wonder how she was going to get my body home if I had died. What a thing to put my mom through! I think about that. It hits home when I hear things like that, from the people that loved me. It was all because I was being selfish. I picked food. Nobody forced that food in me. Nobody forced me to eat all that junk. Nobody forced me to drink all that pop. I did all that to myself. It was very, very selfish of me.

After all those years, selfish years when I was so obese that I couldn't help others, I still wanted to help people, but I felt too restricted to do anything for others, or myself. It's like all that weight was a cage put over me, prison bars I put over myself. I couldn't go out and do things for people because I was insecure, worried about how awful I looked or felt, feeling their stares, the disdain of others gawking at the massive guy. Now that the weight's off I'm free, I can go and do anything to help others, to really live, because what's the point of living if you can't go out and help your fellow man.

Now, I really want to get my head out of the sand and go help others. Nobody cares what you have in your bank account when you die. Nobody cares about what kind of house you have. What people remember is if that person loved them, if they made them smile, helped them or cared for them. That leaves an impression that lasts. I truly believe you can enjoy life to the fullest by giving to other people.

When that switch was thrown inside my head, and I said, "That's enough!" I could add the word "selfishness" right there. "That's enough… selfishness", or that's enough self pity, that's enough feeling sorry for myself. That's enough of being alone. That's enough looking to food for happiness. That's enough of lying to myself.

I've been given a wonderful life. I've truly been blessed! I have a good job. After all my years of obesity, it's a miracle that I stayed as healthy as I did with all that weight. I was blessed that way. I was blessed with loving parents. I'm blessed with good friends that looked past my size, those who just saw me for my heart. I was given all of that, and I was throwing it all away. To me, that could be the biggest problem, the biggest sin there is, because there are people in this world that would long to have the life that I had; the life that I have today. I was throwing it all away, because I was handicapping myself with my size.

The potential that I had was being wasted because of the weight that I chose to carry. That's not smart; throwing away a gift, throwing away everything that many people would kill for. That fire, the Fort McMurray wild fire of May 2016 saved my life. It's sad that after everything that was going on, it took that tragedy for that switch to go off in my head. It took something that extreme happening.

The Blame Game

I don't ever want to be that guy that is looking for someone else to blame. It's not always the other person's fault. I must own it and say sometimes, "This is totally my fault." I want to be kind and understanding, but I don't like how everyone wants to blame the government, blame big business, blame global warming, blame some nation across the seas, blame a political party, blame the media; it seems we all want to blame somebody or something for whatever is wrong in our lives.

I don't blame others. I did it. I was wrong. Sometimes I'll hear a person say, "My spouse is saying this or that to me, making me feel lousy and so *that* is why I'm overeating."

Really? Can someone really put on excess weight because of somebody else's words? I honestly believe very differently, so I would say to that person, "I hear what you're saying, I'm sorry you have been hurt, but still, YOU are the only one that's putting that food in your mouth."

I know there are lots of reasons people struggle with drugs and alcohol, but I have a problem when I hear someone say, "I'm married and my spouse is putting me down, making me feel worthless, so I'm just going to get drunk every night." It's only that person who is the one putting the beer in their own mouth. Ultimately it's our own responsibility, what we do to our own bodies. Nobody's putting a gun to our head to make us eat or drink. The blame game, to me, is just *excuses*.

It's just an excuse to act and behave in a way that gives me an excuse to get away with bad behaviour. It is still, ultimately, our own responsibility. I was 337 pounds heavier, totally because I was out of control with junk food, deep-fried, fast food, burgers, chicken, ice cream, cookies, donuts, the whole mess of it. I was fat because it was my fault. 100% it was my fault. I'm glad I can admit that. It is a big step in getting myself out of this prison cage I built for myself. It's no one's fault except mine.

I'm a big proponent of "self-responsibility". Sure, there were contributing factors; even though I was dealing with loneliness, anger or insecurity, I didn't have to eat all that food. There were healthier ways to deal with it that I didn't chose. There's all kinds of people that are lonely that don't go and eat themselves into an early grave. I could visit any local coffee shop and talk to dozens of people right now that are dealing with worse things than I've ever dealt with, but they didn't turn to booze or food or drugs to deal with it.

I believe that I must be responsible for my own actions in life. I had to come to a point where I wanted to do something about it. I can't stress it enough, "We get one kick at this. That's it." It goes by quickly, like a warm summer breeze, it's here and then it's gone. How do we want to live our one chance? Do I want to be 67 years old, still hanging on to the issues that happened to me when I was in my twenties? Do I want to be using that for an excuse to drink, or eat, or do drugs? Or do I want to get out and enjoy my life? I don't want to be the blame guy. I want to get out there and enjoy the rest of my life. Seriously.

Since I've been given this new lease on life I have come to realize that there's beauty in everything. If I can find the financial means to travel, then I want to travel. If I don't, then I'll go for a walk to the park nearby in my town, or I will drive a few blocks away and check out another park or a new walking trail I've never tried before.

There are nice things to enjoy every day, it doesn't matter if you're poor or rich. My social standing, my job, my clothes or the condo I live in will NOT determine my contentment, or my level of joy and peace. That's why, for me, taking responsibility for myself is a huge deal. I don't blame anybody for anything in my past; all the weight was something I put on. It was all my own fault. I want to be free from that kind of blame game thinking.

We are presented with choices every day. I could have broccoli, or I could have French Fries. I chose French Fries for fourteen years. I could have a salad, or I could have a ten-piece bucket from KFC. I took the bucket for a couple of decades. Those are simply selfish choices. No matter what we do in life, whatever choices we make, there are consequences for those choices. Obviously, if it's a good choice we make, we have good consequences; bad choices yield bad consequence. "A man reaps what he sows."

People might not like me saying this: For me, being almost six hundred pounds, being that size, it was nobody's fault but my own. There was no thyroid issue, no hereditary issue that that would have caused me to get to almost 600 pounds. The only thing that causes people to get up to almost 600 pounds is taking the hand with unhealthy food in it and putting it up to that mouth. That's it. If people combine that with not using their two feet and moving their body from one place to another, that's all it takes. That's what causes obesity. That's what caused me to be 567 pounds.

I can't speak to other issues, and this might come across as being over the top. People might be upset, "how can you say that?" I *can* say it because I lived it. You don't get to be that size unless you're eating unhealthy, crappy food all the time, repeatedly. It has little to do with it being hereditary and it has very little to do with the thyroid. Those might account for maybe ten, twenty or thirty pounds, sure. Could an extra 337 pounds on my body be caused by genetics? No way! Not in my case.

That's how I was raised. My mom and dad were very giving. Newfoundland people themselves are very generous. Canadians are some of the kindest, most gracious people in the world. If you don't agree with me, I have to say, "Sorry!"

I found out one thing for sure through the fire and evacuation, that Canada is an incredibly giving and supportive nation. Each province has its little quirks. Alberta might make fun of Saskatchewan, Saskatchewan might tease their friends from Manitoba, P.E.I. and New Brunswick might have a rivalry in curling, but we know for sure that when a country's facing a national disaster, everybody comes together. Edmonton and Calgary have always been deeply competitive, but when people from Fort McMurray were being evacuated those two cities came together to help evacuees in an instant in one concerted effort.

My parents, growing up in that small little town in northern Newfoundland, never had much. Nobody really had much, but you could knock on the door of any house in my little town and say, "Hi, my name is Bob and I'm really hungry, I need something to eat." I don't think a single home in that whole town would turn anyone away.

That's the way it should be. I was raised in a Christian household, with Christian values, with the Bible, with Jesus' life as an example, all having this same message in common: we're here on this planet to love others, to love God and to give, even sacrificially. Jesus didn't have to come down to this earth. He was royalty. He gave it all up. That's how I was brought up. My stuff doesn't mean a thing to me. Things don't mean a thing to me. Nice cars, nice homes; it's nice to be comfortable. I have a comfortable life. That doesn't mean a thing to me. What means something to me is what's inside a guys' heart. I have wonderful Muslim friends, I have wonderful Christian friends, I have wonderful friends that don't believe in any religion, but they'll give you the shirt off their back. When it comes down to it, that's how we are meant to live life regardless of our upbringing.

We all need each other. There's no greater joy in this world than being able to help one another, especially when we don't look for anything, or want anything in return. When I can give to somebody anonymously, without any credit, without telling people what I've done, that's how and who I want to be. I want to help people, to be that guy who goes into a restaurant and secretly pays for a stranger's meal; to never let them know who paid for it.

I feel like I've lost a lot in the past fourteen years, not being able to do that, being so limited by my size and the insecurities that went with it. The world's a beautiful place. There's a lot of hurting people out there that don't need much. They just want somebody to know that somebody cares, that there's hope. That's why I hope, somebody can read this, somebody can see this and be inspired to change, to grow and to get free.

No Longer a Slave

This next part has been huge for me. In the past couple years since my life has changed, I'm very aware of the theme of "freedom". It's truly a powerful concept. Abraham Lincoln was a pivotal character in history because he knew how important freedom was. The same is true of Martin Luther King Jr. It was his life's goal to enter eternity and life in racially oppressed America declaring "Free at last, free at last. Thank God Almighty, I'm free at last."

I never really knew that I was walking around every single day of my life in a prison cell. Obviously, it wasn't a prison with bars and chains, a spring bed and mattress, a concrete box with a swinging metal door and a toilet in the corner. My prison looked different. It was a prison of flesh; 337 extra pounds of it to be exact. In the last chapter I talked about what it was like being a prisoner, but now, let me focus on what it was like becoming free!

I was talking with a buddy the other day about making some travel plans next month and this idea just popped up as we were talking, saying that when I'm in Toronto being interviewed on CTV for their national morning news show, I think I might just head down to Cancun afterwards. I have a connection down there and flights are cheap from Toronto. I might just do that. I can't believe I can say or think of stuff like that! I feel like a rock star or something. "I think I'll just fly to Mexico next month for a few days." Who says stuff like that? Free people do!

I make a good salary from my work. Now that I'm easily spending $500 per month LESS on food, transitioning from junk food to normal groceries, I have more spare cash. Now that I don't have to drive to work every day and can take the bus for free, I'm probably saving another $500 per month on gas. It's not uncommon to go three weeks without having to put gas in my car. I have more money, plus I have more stamina, need less sleep. Guess what? I can take more overtime shifts now, easily and not be in pain! I can't believe the difference this lifestyle change has made financially for me!

It wasn't the money that held me back from taking a break before. It was the restriction of not being able to fit in an airplane seat. I couldn't get the seat belt on. Even with the seat belt extension, I still couldn't get the seat belt on. It always felt tight, crowded. I couldn't go to that tiny little bathroom (truth be told, I still can't, it's just really small in there). Then, if I did get there they might not have a car rental big enough for me, or a hotel shuttle that I could fit into. There were countless things that restricted me from travelling. It felt like I was in prison.

Now, I can take off anywhere, anytime. I can go almost anywhere in the world! Do you get what I'm saying? Do you understand what a HUGE deal this is for me? Are you picking up what I'm laying down? I'm free. I can do whatever I want. That's why I feel like a rock star!

I love that freedom. I have been at this weight for almost a year now and I'm still smiling about it. I don't think I will ever stop smiling about this. If there's anything I still can't get over, the greatest excitement with this entire change of lifestyle journey, it's the freedom. Just freedom. I'm not slowed down by my body anymore. I'm not constricted in a world that is *not* designed for obese people. I can enjoy the world like an average-sized person. I'm free.

If I get on a plane, nobody looks at me any differently or with judgement in their eyes. I can sit down in the seat like any normal person would without assistance or special seating arrangements or a seat belt extension. It's almost unbelievable to me. I can walk down the centre aisle of the plane and nobody says, "Oh, there's a big guy coming." I'm the guy looking at them now. When I hear the term "big guy", I wonder who they're talking about? I get in my seat, put my armrest down, put my tray table down and there's all kinds of room. It's freedom!

Now there are NO restrictions. I am enjoying and appreciating this freedom so much that I could wake up tomorrow morning and if the bank came and took everything, I'd be fine. I'd still be smiling. It wouldn't get me down and it wouldn't bother me a bit. They could take it all, because I've got my health and I'm truly free to do anything now. You know, once you've got your health and the freedom that goes with it, you've got everything you need. I could start over time and time again. I can do whatever it is I've got to do to survive. I can do anything, not only can I travel, I am now liberated to do whatever I want. I have freedom of movement. It's such a simple thing, but I had been in jail surrounded by 337 pounds of excess body weight that slowly grew on my body for about twenty years.

I don't have to worry about anxiety issues just trying to buy clothes. I don't have to worry about people staring at me, judging me. I don't have to worry about fitting into any vehicle.

I don't have to worry about going to a restaurant and having a table instead of a booth.

I remember, one time, I went to the Keg in Edmonton. I asked the hostess for a table. She brought me to the table, but at the table, there were these rickety little chairs with flimsy little arms. For a guy my size, it was way too small. As I was sitting there in this feeble, pathetic chair, I was wedged in there really good, well, actually, just the back third of my butt was in the chair with a lot of my weight on my two feet and using a portion of my butt on that chair as the third part of a tripod. It was awful. That was the only way I could sit. The waitress came to the table to check on my meal and I know she had good intentions, but she brought a sturdier chair without arms on it and she said, "Excuse me, sir. Would you like this chair? This is one we keep for pregnant women." I wanted to bury my head in the sand. I already had my meal there. If not for that, I would have gotten up and walked out.

Many embarrassing moments like that happened, shameful, humiliating moments. Now, seating is a non-issue; it's nothing. I still smile every time I sit in a restaurant. Like the other day I was in Calgary and before I sat down at Tim Hortons I had to smile. They have those fixed seats like they do in any fast food restaurant with the swivel chairs at the little tables. Before, I could never fit into those seats but now I just slide in and there is all kinds of room. It's all those little details that just make me smile, everyday. Just three short years ago, I never, ever thought I would see this. I never thought any of this would be possible. I didn't think I'd see 45 year of age!

I'm loving life so much now! I'm totally enjoying the freedom. The *freedom*; that's the word that describes it all. The freedom I now have, all that junk I ate stole from me. There's not a chance I would ever let that happen again. I have freedom. I left behind all the lies that junk food told me, lies of happiness and what it was really doing.

Free from Fear

Health Fear — I used to have another friend, Mark Baker. If he didn't hear from me for a few days, he would give me a call or come over to the house if he couldn't reach me. He was always afraid I was going to be dead with a heart attack, and nobody would know. I had the same fear.

I've had my heart checked and everything's great. No signs of stress or damage or anything! Nothing! Let me say again, I think the only way that I came through all of this with no serious problems is because of the prayers of my mom. Seriously. To think that I survived years in that big body is nothing short of a miracle. The only thing I suffer from sometimes is low blood pressure!

The doctor checked for diabetes in the beginning of my weight loss, because I thought I had it, because I was getting all this tingling sensation down my legs and eye issues. When the bloodwork came back she said there was nothing there. No diabetes, no problems.

I think of all those risky times taking chances out on the highway, driving in the wintertime in northern Alberta in the snow, in 20 degree below conditions or worse. What if I would have lost control and gone in the ditch? I hate to think of it. If I would have gotten hurt, there's no stretcher big enough to hold me. How would they have ever gotten me out of a front-end collision. The air bag would have hit me and just gone straight up and then forward to the windshield. There was no room for it to go anywhere else. All that driving into work in poor conditions. Something could have happened, but nothing ever happened. I was always afraid that it would have.

Being jumbo sized I realize I was also at a greater risk of cancer. However, probably my biggest health concern was slipping and falling and maybe breaking something. In the wintertime, if I fell and broke my leg, broke my foot, if I broke anything I would have been in huge trouble. It's bad enough being that size, there is a terrible lack of mobility. Add to that, trying to get through the day just being able to move. I could barely move as it was. With something broken, I wouldn't be able to get a wheel chair big enough to hold my weight. Where would I get crutches strong enough? Cast iron crutches would be too heavy to lift. There's nothing designed to help people at that size.

Getting sick or injured was a fear that I lived with constantly. This will sound odd, but I was so happy last summer, when I got sick, and very thankful, because, with the weight gone, it was all manageable. They were able to do surgery and get me fixed up with no complications. To be put on a plane, to have to fly to another city or travel 7 or 8 hours in an ambulance to get into a hospital room that could accommodate my 567 pounds? Wow. That would have been terrible. As it turned out, I got to have the surgery and resolve those medical issues at a local hospital.

I'm not afraid of health issues any more.

Family Fears — I used to worry about what would happen, God forbid, if mom or dad died, how would I get home? Mom and dad are up there in age, so, it's possible. I could fly home, but I would have had to buy two seats. That would cost a lot of money. Then when the plane lands in Deer Lake, what car do I rent to get up home? There's probably not a lot of full-size rentals at that airport. My mother has a little Toyota Corolla, that won't fit me. My brother had a Dodge truck, that didn't even fit me when I was heavy. How could I get home? What do I do when I am home? There's no public transit, no Uber, no jumbo taxi's, no way to get around in that little town.

All of these fears used to plague my mind constantly. Not a day would go by that I wouldn't be thinking about these fears and having anxiety. Then on top of the normal day to day problems of life, I was dealing with all of these issues alone. Now I can go see my family any time. I can rent a car or get picked up in any car. It's no problem.

Fear of Dying Alone — I'm not just talking now about being lonely, but this fear that could end up being crippling, it was a two-fold fear. 1. The fear of dying and, 2. the fear of dying alone. The fear of dying alone was bad because I used to think, well, here I am, the rest of my life, living up in Fort McMurray, in the middle of nowhere, my family are mostly far away. If I die alone in that condo, no one's going to find me for like three or four days until I'm due at my next work shift. What kind of messy impact is that going to have on my daughter? My parents? My brother?

The fear of dying? I'll be the first to admit, I haven't always clung to my faith as close as I would have liked. I've followed God, but I've been distant at times. I've gotten away from Him quite a few times, but He's never gotten away from me, He's never left me. I remember times, I'd be in the tire shop at work. I'd be driving a piece of equipment and go get a tire, and I would know God was with me. I'd sense His gentle presence or I would feel something in my mind, I'd feel something quietly tugging at my heart, trying to love me, trying to help me.

I'd always know that even if I wasn't in a perfect place where I should be, conscious of God, in tune with Him, He was still with me. There was a calling on my life, a sense of calling to serve in a church, in ministry, and I never really felt that I had fulfilled that. Sometimes a part of me wonders if, maybe because I felt like I was running from God, like the bible story of Jonah, maybe I had missed it, maybe I was cursed a little bit. It felt like I was always alone, always single, always wanted to have a family but never did fully have a wife and kids. Then the weight issues crept in. To me that unshakable tension in my heart of being stuck where I was at, not really embracing all that God had for my life, living up to my potential, losing the weight with God's help, it seemed like sometimes I was cursed and I often wondered if this was what is was like, how Cain felt.

God was there, I believe that God was always there. I just wasn't connecting with Him, I was not spending time with God or being with God. He was there, but I was avoiding Him. I suspect many of you know what I'm talking about. He's following you and me, He loves us, He's right there, but, He's also gently knocking on the door of our heart, whispering to us, believing in us, believing for something better for us, hoping for us, challenging us, reminding me that "this is not where you're supposed to be sonny. I didn't bring you this far only to have you changing tires in Northern Alberta your whole life" but, I think, I know He has provided this job for me. I believe *that* to this day. I think God loves me and He loves you and He has a wonderful plan for our lives.

I don't think things happen by chance. I don't think Emma was an accident in my life and this incredible story of my life with her isn't a fluke, but I honestly do believe, that God has great plans for all of us.

Things really sucked for me. God helped me turn it all around. Now I get to talk to all kinds of people and encourage them and help them. The things that were destroying my life, well, unbelievably I have bounced back from tragedy to triumph. It's amazing. I attribute it to God being overwhelmingly kind to me. It's not because I'm so special. The bible actually tells us that God didn't give us an attitude or a mindset of fear, but an attitude of love, of power (or capability) and the ability to be self-controlled or a soundness of mind (2 Timothy 1:7). I'm not trying to be preachy here, this is just who I am. My faith in God keeps bubbling up to the surface in my story. I must give credit where credit is due. God has given me a praying mom and the strength to turn this all around. He really loves you too. He wants to help you too. Just invite Him, you don't need some fancy prayer or religious ceremony, just talk to Him. He's right there with you right now. Seriously. Why not ask for His help?

I always feel Him near, He comforts me. You can feel him too! This might sound funny, but it's kind of like a Slinky. You can stretch that Slinky out and you can be on the other end miles away from God, but he's still attached at the other end. Every once in a while the slinky is stretched as far as it can go, He springs back and bangs right up against you. You feel him right close. You might try to run away, just living life without God and you stretch that Slinky again then boom, He's right there again. He's never far away.

Again, I'm not saying I'm anything special, but I am totally thrilled that doing this crazy change of lifestyle thing has given me a huge platform to tell hundreds and hundreds of people, actually thousands, actually over a million people have viewed the original CBC News story online — and I have the privilege of telling you all that you are not alone.

You. Are. Not. Alone.

Almost the entirety of this book (the 1st Edition anyways) has been written and developed in December of 2018. It's really neat to be putting this together while the Christmas carols are playing and some of the songs mention this one particular name of Jesus: Emmanuel. That name literally means "God with us." I'm glad to write this and encourage you with my story. I can relate to you, whatever your addiction, however huge your pain might be, I can relate. I've known pain, shame, guilt, worthlessness, the whole gamut of negative emotions. I want to encourage you that you're not alone. Even better than that thought is the fact that God who created the universe wants you to know that you are not alone and He loves you and wants to bless you and help you and turn your life around into the greatest possible version of who He has created you to be.

"CAN anything ever separate us from God's love? Does it mean He no longer loves us if we have trouble or calamity, or are persecuted, or hungry, or destitute, or in danger, or threatened with death?

No, despite all these things, overwhelming victory is ours through Christ, who loved us.

And I am convinced that nothing can ever separate us from God's love. Neither death nor life, neither angels nor demons, neither our fears for today nor our worries about tomorrow--not even the powers of hell can separate us from God's love.

No power in the sky above or in the earth below--indeed, nothing in all creation will ever be able to separate us from the love of God that is revealed in Christ Jesus our Lord."

— St. Paul the Apostle

(Romans 8:35, 37-39, NLT)

I'm not afraid of dying. I will never be alone. I'm not worried about dying alone. That's not possible.

7

First Steps

I like to be really practical. I have gone to great lengths in the previous chapter to talk about my changes in thinking and attitude, but let me continue with my story.

This Is My Chance!

I have always been the type of guy who tries to find the positive in everything. When I found myself evacuated as part of the largest evacuation in Canadian history, even though I stayed positive a part of me was crying out, "This is it! If I don't do it this time, there might not be another chance."

When you're clinically obese there is always that possibility that you're walking a fine line between life and death; literally any moment it could be all over. I certainly believe I was at that point. I had often wondered if I would have a massive heart attack, keel over and die right on the spot. I had chest pains before. The thought that there might not be any more chances may have been very accurate. Who knows? It might have truly been my last chance to change that day on the bus, the plane arriving in Edmonton and going for supper. That could have been the night a triple cheeseburger would have killed me.

When I got to Edmonton, I drove to the suburb of St. Albert that first night of the second evacuation and immediately things changed. I think my first meal was at Swiss Chalet. Before that evening, I would order the double leg chicken dinner, a side of fries, a dessert of pecan pie warmed up with ice-cream on the side, a pop with the meal, and maybe an extra plate of fries. Of course I'd have the Chalet Sauce and a roll or two, maybe three.

After that switch went off in my head, I remember sitting there thinking, "What's the healthiest way I can do this?" In that moment, and now when I go to Swiss Chalet, I still get a double leg chicken dinner, but instead of fries I get the veggies. That's all! At Swiss Chalet the vegetables are usually broccoli, cauliflower and carrots, a mixed vegetable option; no gravy, no fries, no bread and just like that, it's a very healthy meal. When the chicken would land at the table, I'd just take off the skin, and I'd have a glass of water, not a Diet Pepsi.

I knew that something must have changed, because before when I would try to diet or change things, I would order a couple of healthy meals, but the urges for junk food would just overtake me. I would just give up within a day or two. This time it was different, because although the urges were still there, even though the cravings were still there and I still *really* wanted a bag of chips and a caramel ice cream cone, like you wouldn't believe… I kept thinking, *"This is enough. I can't keep doing this. I have to change. I'm not getting younger, I'm not getting smaller by any means. I'm done with all that. Enough!"*

When I went into restaurants, which I did quite a bit being evacuated, I would order healthy options. That's another thing I have to point out here: people make excuses, "Well, I'm traveling, so I have to eat out a lot, so I can't diet. I have to be on the road with my job. I have to eat in who-knows-what-restaurant, so it's hard to watch what I eat." That's bull crap! Of course you can eat healthy if you choose to eat healthy! You can go into any restaurant and pick a healthy option. Even as recently as ordering when we went out to eat last night. I had a bowl of soup and a salad. I didn't get the nachos, no deep-fried appetizers, no piece of pie for dessert, I just chose a healthy soup and salad. It was delicious!

I haven't been perfect with it. Maybe some of the sauces or salad dressings could be better, but I'm picking the healthiest options there are on the menu. I'm always getting vegetables, I'm ordering soup, I'm choosing a salad over meat and potatoes consistently. If I have meat, I'll choose a lower fat option, I'll throw out the chicken skin. I choose veggies over potatoes. I might have some rice, but not bread or fries. I always take the healthiest option that I can find. When I go to Tony Roma's for example, I'd love to have the ribs, but I scan the menu, and the best thing I know of there is what I always get at Tony Roma's; the salmon with veggies, and a side of rice. That's a beautiful healthy meal. There are no excuses. If I lost my first thirty pounds (or maybe more) living in a hotel for just over three weeks, having to eat out just about every day, if I can do it, anybody can.

A lot of it comes down to how badly you want it. Everything in life is a choice. You can choose a healthy meal at a restaurant, or you can choose high carb, greasy, fatty fast food. It's your call. I just did what I knew.

Not Rocket Science

I still don't know the science behind a lot of it. I'm learning quite a bit about what I'm doing and why it works as I go along. When I started, all I knew was being the size I was, anything was better than what I was eating. As soon as I gave my body a little bit of help it was almost like it hugged me back and said, "Thanks! Let's get the ball rolling now." Compared to what I used to eat, I was eating more vegetables than I ever did before which was a wonderful healthy adjustment. I considered potatoes to be my vegetable before and usually French fried. I had so few vegetables, it's a wonder I never got scurvy like the old explorers on the seas hundreds of years ago.

As I arrived in Red Deer, I realized, "I can't go into work right now, my whole town has been evacuated. I suppose I have an opportunity right now to start changing my lifestyle." I didn't know how long I was going to be off work, how long I was going to be down south in Red Deer, Alberta, about six hours away from home. Why wait to get home to start? I was at a hotel. There was time. There was nothing else to do. I figured, "I have opportunity today to lose weight and I'm not making any more excuses!"

One of my favourite spots in the province of Alberta is Sylvan Lake, a picturesque little holiday town, a short drive from Red Deer. I hoped to take advantage of this quaint little town nearby during this break.

Eastern Alberta is mostly flat prairie and farmland. To the west are the beautiful Canadian Rockies, one of the most beautiful regions in the world. Many parts of the province are a semi-arid climate. In Central Alberta, tucked away between the mountain and prairie extremes, there are a number of lakes like Sylvan. I really like the area. With my family roots in Newfoundland, right on the Atlantic Ocean, I have always loved the water. Alberta doesn't have lots of water like eastern Canada does with lakes everywhere. I would love nothing more than to hop in my car, drive to Sylvan Lake and walk around the water. It was only about a twenty-minute drive from town.

I started, just a few minutes at first, but continued to keep walking more each day. I only walked five minutes the first day, but it nearly killed me. I'd drive over there every day. To be near the joy and comfort of water those first couple weeks, gave me inspiration in that season. That was a positive little thing for me to cling to; being near the water. That was my little slice of heaven; just the sound of water feeds my soul.

I've always been a busy man, or I've kept myself busy at least, even if it was driving around to get a bunch of donuts and sit by the water when I was still heavy. Being in Red Deer, I said to myself, "This is my chance here. I can't go into work right now, so I have to do this, and I have to do it now." I just started walking and changing what I ate, and that was it. That was my new lifestyle.

I could barely walk to my car without getting out of breath. It was very hard. I would get overheated if I walked too quickly, just start sweating and breathing heavy. When I first started walking, I felt like somebody at the bottom of a huge mountain, looking way up to the top. I had started walking or dieting so many times before and I had never succeeded, but something about this seemed different to me. Finally, something just clicked, "I can't keep living my life like this! I just can't do that lazy, junk food thing any more!"

I would still wake up in the morning and see my fat self in the mirror. I'd ask myself, "How am I going to do this? I'm too fat to walk!" but, every day I'd just push myself a little more, a little more. I kept at it, and kept at it. It was very hard. I mean it was **REALLY** hard.

I mentioned earlier the picture of walking around with seven water jugs tying them to your back, 350 extra pounds and then going for a five-minute stroll down by the lake! That's what I mean by *really* hard.

Withdrawal

I was going through withdrawal. Cold turkey does that. There was no more pop. No cases of twenty-four diet sodas to calm my nerves, especially when going through such a hard time like the stress of a major crisis from the wildfires. Being evacuated a couple times is heavy. Not knowing if I was going to have a job to go back to was worrisome. I didn't know what shape our city would be in when we all returned, what our city was going to look like or if there even was going to be a city at all. I wondered if I was going to have a condo to live in and I wondered how long my paycheques would keep coming. My company was wonderful to all of their employees. They kept paying us and giving us benefits even though the operations were shut down! Who does that? Who is kind enough to pay out when nothing was coming in? I still worried how long that would keep going.

It wasn't the ideal time to quit the carbs, the sugar or diet soda addiction, or the caffeine addiction. If I ever "needed" caffeine and sugar, it was right then, during the trauma of the evacuation, the wildfire, the worries and concerns, the ultimate time for an excuse to keep eating and drinking like I had the last 15 or 20 years.

I would get shaky from having no caffeine and no sugar. Headaches? Wow. I can't begin to describe how intense the headaches were coming off of years of sugar, carbs, grease and oil, preservatives, chemicals. God only knows the toxins that were in my system from a lifetime of self-indulgence and self-abuse. I have never done drugs or been a drinker, it's just not my thing, but I have experienced pretty heavy withdrawal symptoms coming off of my food addiction cold turkey.

Those withdrawal symptoms touched other areas: I was cranky a bit because for years I was having a lot of sugar, a lot of pop, a lot of fried foods, a lot of carbs that eventually turn into body fat after I would eat them. I was giving up my only comfort, my best friend, food. I was giving up a lot. At a time when anybody would be very understanding if I put on more weight, "Tony's eating even more, he's all stressed out going through the fire, you have to understand he's under a lot of stress."

Instead, that's the moment I changed my lifestyle and started to lose weight. So even through all the stress and uncertainty, I gave up my dearest addiction, my crutch, my treats, my rewards, my source of comfort and I'm so very glad I did.

I didn't go hide out at a fat farm where every temptation was removed. Those first few weeks, driving out to Sylvan Lake, there were lots of nice little restaurants there all around me, a Dairy Queen, a couple Tim Hortons. The thought entered my head "I've been doing really well. I should just go get a triple-triple and a couple donuts." The temptation would enter my head, but I kept on track thinking "I can't, because that's the same thing I would always do before and it was killing me. It was ruining my life."

Pressing Through

I figured all of this was not going to last forever - this evacuation trip to Red Deer. I didn't know what the future held. I would keep thinking about my future those days. When tragedy or problems happen, people tend to turn to things that make them feel happy, whether that's alcohol, or drugs, or food. My thing was food, obviously. Being down there in Red Deer, staying in a hotel, it's a fairly easy environment to put ON some weight. It's easy to just go to a convenience store, get some potato chips, some chocolate, some ice cream and come back to the comfy hotel and eat myself into oblivion for a couple weeks, but no, not me, not this time. This was my time.

It was still consistently close to 30 degrees Celsius outside.

It was 30 all that month, I remember that month very clearly. As a huge guy I hated those hot spells. Alberta was dusty, it was dry, and there was the smell of smoke all over the province. It was still like a thick haze; the smoke was miserable. I would breathe in, it would be dusty, dry and smoky, even near the lake. As I walked my heart would be pounding, it always was. My head was pounding. My ears would be ringing - I'm sure from my blood pressure being up. My energy level was very low, it was always low, but without the sugar rush, without the diet cola to give me a caffeine kick, it's a wonder I didn't slip into a coma.

I was still walking without socks. I was still walking in the velcro running shoes. I was still walking with my left foot angled to the side. I was still walking in my old 7XL gym pants and an old 6XL, stained t-shirt. It wasn't easy. It wasn't pretty. It wasn't glamorous. Something had clicked. Something inside me said, "This is enough". I had to push through and get it done.

I felt very drained, those first few weeks, but I'd feel I would survive because I was by the water. Water always has a way of bringing peace to me. I love the ocean. I love a big lake, or an ocean. There's just something about hearing those waves roll in, it just seems to wash away all my problems. It didn't of course, I was still terribly overweight; but I chose to focus on that little bit of positive. Believe me, those first three weeks were NOT happy.

It was hard physically, but it was also tough emotionally because all my "happiness" go-to's were now gone. No more "treats". There was no going back and having a bag of chips, or going for a drive to pick up a donut or two, or grabbing an ice cream bar or a cone. All that was gone. I don't drink, I don't smoke, so I didn't have anything to fall back on. It was rough.

I was in the beginning stages of losing weight, but I was still huge. There were no immediate rewards or pay offs. I was just perpetually miserable.

I wish I could say the moment I started to change my lifestyle, things were great, but really, they were pretty awful for those first few weeks. There was also some emotional baggage being an evacuee, being displaced from home. I needed something. Some little thing or things to keep me going; something other than ice cream or fried chicken or French Fries or other unhealthy choices. After I would walk, I loved going for a relaxing drive. So, I would grab a coffee, without three sugars and three creams, just black or with half a cream, and I'd go for a drive and explore. That little innocent pleasure, seeing Emma and enjoying the water was all I had.

Sometimes I'd bring Emma along for my walks or drives to the lake. I was very thankful that I got to spend more time with her while I was in Red Deer. I'd drive her to school, I'd pick her up. Those were, really, my only little positive reinforcements; spending time with Emma, going for drives and enjoying walks along Sylvan Lake with a coffee. It was just enough to keep me going.

Those initial walks were very painful. My heart was racing, everything was either jiggling or in pain, but I kept pushing myself. Even those five minutes that first day felt like a marathon in 30+ degree heat, six minutes the next day felt like Hell, but I steadily kept pushing.

I kept doing that; kept right at the walking. I kept eating healthy. Honestly, I had doubts even myself if I would stay with it, because when I tried dieting before it never stuck, but something was different this time. My thinking was different. I didn't need a break. I didn't need a treat. I was sick of where that was leading. I just kept at it, and kept at it.

As each day would go by, I'd push myself a bit farther. Five minutes soon became ten minutes, which soon turned into fifteen minutes. The first time I walked a half hour straight I was overjoyed. It took me three weeks to hit that goal, and being at a hotel, I had no access to a scale, but, it felt good to hit a time target. I was finding out details every now and then of what was going on with the fire, and how people were hearing the news of loss and the stress was bombarding all of us evacuees regularly.

I found the walking really helped me mentally and emotionally. It helped me clear my head and relax. I would do a lot of thinking as I walked, I'd even process my thoughts out loud sometimes, talking to myself a bit.

Fort McMurray remained under the mandatory evacuation order for almost a month. The highway through town was open, but only to go through town, not into town. Every side street was closed off the highway. There was limited gas available north of Wandering River, so commuters needed to ensure enough gas in their vehicle for a return trip because everything in Fort McMurray was still closed. Everything. Citizens were finally allowed back into Fort McMurray in early June, I think I went back June the 10th. As we were allowed back into the city, driving into Fort McMurray the destruction was obvious and widespread; It was a solemn thing.

When the news came that we were allowed back into Fort McMurray, it was a great relief for all of us. It was a relief for us residents and for a province that had hosted us very kindly and graciously. I'm sure it was also a huge sigh of relief for the firefighters and other first responders who had battled the blaze and the many professionals who got electricity and other essential services back online.

From my understanding, I think it was over 3200 structures that were destroyed; homes and businesses. With just under $4 Billion in insurance claims, the Fort McMurray wildfire was the most expensive disaster in Canadian history. About 10% of Fort McMurray residents lost their homes. Many neighbourhoods, businesses and industries were destroyed, but miraculously, no one was killed as a direct result of the fire.

It was an incredibly cool and even ironic moment that when the mandatory evacuation was lifted. Highway 63 opened to allow cars back into the city (not just through the city). On top of one of the overpasses two fire trucks with those huge extension ladders hoisted a giant Canadian flag with an Alberta flag and a Fort McMurray flag on either side to welcome the residents back home. Along the side of the bridge was another banner that read "We support Fort McMurray". Those fire fighters who had risked their lives to save and protect our city were the first to welcome us back. It was a proud moment that made national and even international news.

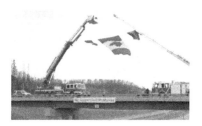

Fort McMurray firefighters proudly display Canada, Alberta and Civic flags over highway 63 as residents return home following weeks of mandatory evacuation.

Driving back through the outskirts of the city, it was painful to see all the burnt trees; destroyed businesses and homes. Entire neighbourhoods were totally burned down, still cordoned off, with no one allowed in. Those scenes, those memories still stick in my mind. Those wildfires really impacted our town.

I drove towards my neighbourhood in the north end of town. I was very, very fortunate. My condo was untouched by fire. There was some smoke damage, pretty much everywhere in the city, but I never even lost power, my fridge was still running when I got home. There were several parts of the city, in neighbourhoods not far from where I lived, there were entire areas, like 20 or 30 houses in one spot burned to the ground; people's homes, everything gone. All over the roads there were cars and trucks burnt out.

Some areas were not only burned down, but they had already bulldozed the area and knocked the remnants down to make fire breaks. Where there used to be parks, nice forested areas sections of it were all just flattened, bulldozed down to keep the fires from coming close to the homes that remained. It felt like we were coming home into a war zone.

The air quality was still poor, and the smoke lingered. I have seen pictures of maps where the smoke went, covering southern Alberta and heading into Central Canada, all the way up to northern Quebec and even Labrador. The smoke travelled through the Central U.S. all the way to Texas and all of Florida. It had a huge impact on the continent.

After a few weeks residents were allowed to go into certain areas and just look around. I realized how fortunate I was to still have my place, but I felt really horrible for many friends and co-workers who lost homes. I had one friend, he lost his dogs, his house, everything. He was very close to his pets. That was hard for him. That loss was like losing a family member.

It's amazing to see how strong people are too! Some people that I know lost everything, but they were saying, "I still have my health. I look at my home, it's only stuff." I admire their strength, but still, it's sad to hear those stories.

For most people, insurance covered the cost of their home or business being replaced. The town has been rebuilt and has recovered very well. However, it's not uncommon to hear of people that are still dealing with insurance issues; even to this day, two and a half years after the fire. Housing prices have dropped considerably. Fort McMurray used to be one of the most expensive cities to live in Canada. Now the housing prices have dropped significantly. We have all taken a big hit in that way.

My insurance company, AMA, was wonderful to me. I feel bad for some people who didn't do as well as I did with insurance. If you drive around Fort McMurray even today, there are big signs on some houses complaining, "Never buy insurance from…" some company listed on the sign, two and a half years later. It's really sad.

From my understanding, there are people that opted to file for bankruptcy. A lot of people never came back. Fort McMurray's a very resilient town, a very strong community. It's been through a lot with the oil downturn; there have been many booms and busts over the years. There were many infrastructure issues during the boom years; they couldn't get enough homes up quickly enough.

These days, international oil prices are low so we're still having an oil crisis; but Fort McMurray people remain strong. There are lots of news stories about pipelines not being built and we currently have a backlog of oil needing to be shipped out, but Fort McMurray stays strong. Fort McMurray people have always been strong and determined people, very caring and giving. It's a wonderful city. I love Fort McMurray. It's my home. It's getting rebuilt very quickly. It's a beautiful family town; lots of parks, community centres, shops and restaurants. There's everything in Fort McMurray you'd ever need in a city. It'll keep bouncing back. It always does.

We were very fortunate that the fires never got to the water treatment plant. The fires never burned the hospital. If it got either of those two things, goodness knows how long it would have taken before we were allowed back. None of the major utility central operations were touched either, we lost many electrical poles and telephone lines, but those were rebuilt quickly.

When we got back to town, it was kind of surreal because they still didn't have the hospital open. They had hospital services set up on the hospital grounds in a bunch of army tents, like a MASH unit. They were doing hospital work there. They still had to clean the hospital before they could re-open. In fact, every building, every school, every business and every office in Fort McMurray had to be cleaned. The grocery stores all had to be cleaned. As I understand, all of that food had to be thrown out. Basically, the whole city had to be cleaned.

At my condo building, relatively untouched, we never lost power, but everything had to be cleaned. There was soot and smoke damage everywhere. Leaving in an emergency evacuation protocol, when I did get around to leaving, I didn't think to check everything and in the middle of the confusion, I had left a window open! I thought for sure I was going to have a ton of smoke damage. There was some smoke damage, but it wasn't really too bad. I was thankful.

There was one very unusual thing that we saw on TV and heard on the radio and we were warned about. They were saying, since a lot of people had lost power, they were warning us, "Do not open your fridge." After a month without power, the meats and everything else perishable without refrigeration had began to rot. What a nightmare! They said, "If you lost power, just duct tape your fridge shut and put it out by the curb. Do not attempt to open it or clean it out."

It took a while, but all of those dead, moldy, filthy fridges were duct taped shut, picked up and taken away. Driving around town, everywhere in the city, you would see all of these fridges at the side of the road; with duct tape on them. Some of the fridges had hockey tape keeping them shut. This is Canada after all, and people do run out of duct tape.

I was also very lucky that the one thing I did remember to

do before I left was take the garbage out. Garbage was a huge issue in the weeks following the fire, and then there were flies and millions of wasps after a few weeks, reinforcing our feeling of the apocalypse or at least the ten plagues of biblical proportions. I didn't have an issue with flies or wasps or hornets as so many Fort McMurray residents did in those weeks. I was lucky that way. I thought to take the garbage out, but I didn't have the sense to close the window with smoke everywhere outside!

When I came back, I cleaned my place out, and I kept up my diet. Not long after that, I went back to work. When I got back to work, I was in for one of the greatest shocks of my life when I found out how much weight I had lost. I knew it was a rough few weeks eating well and walking but I felt I was making progress. I had eaten no sugar, no carbs, no bread, no pasta, no potatoes; just meat and vegetables and some fruit. I had consistently kept walking every day, sometimes twice a day, despite of the pain and misery and my grumbling.

I had increased my daily walking a minute or two each day so that by the end of three weeks of being away I had gotten up to walking 30 minutes at a time. Thirty minutes! Do you understand what a big deal that was? In former days, I used to alter my terrible diet so I would not have to go to the bathroom at work because it was "too far" to walk a few minutes to the other building to use the larger bathroom stalls? That I would be out of breath for taking that little walk? And now I was walking 30 minutes a day? It was a proud moment for me to break that barrier.

I remember the first time I did a half hour walk. I texted my work buddy, Anas. I think he was just getting back from Morocco, where he spent the evacuation. He was over there during the fire. He was very proud of me, and to be honest, I was proud of me too!

When I finally got to work, in June of 2016, the first day back I used the industrial scale at work, the one that could hold my weight (unlike the scales I had ruined at work). I normally broke any bathroom scale I stepped on because I was too big. There was, however, that scale at work big enough to hold me and the last time I had stepped on it, before the fires, I was 567 pounds. No other scale would hold me.

I wasn't sure if there would be any improvement, but I knew it would be the same scale so I would have an accurate tool to measure my progress. This was the scale that measured me at one of my heaviest weights ever. My weight may have been higher than 567, even quite a bit higher, but that was the scale that had measured my weight about four months before the evacuation.

So, I weighed myself and for the first time in over twenty years, my weight had gone down. I had lost thirty pounds!

Twenty years earlier when I was in College, I went on a diet and lost some weight. That was when I was in my 20's. To my knowledge I had not lost a pound since then. I had only continually gotten heavier for two decades.

When I read the 537 number on the scale, I actually didn't believe it. I got off the scale twice and re-weighed myself because I saw something I had never seen before, not since college. For the majority of my life I had constantly put on the weight little by little, ever since I was born. But now…?

MY WEIGHT HAD GONE DOWN. Down!? No, it couldn't be. There must have been some kind of problem or malfunction, but then after the third time on the scale, with the exact same result each time I had stepped on, I knew it was true. My weight had gone *DOWN!!!*

It was like a dream. It was too good to be true, but it was true. Thirty pounds were gone. Thirty pounds! I know that is only 5% of my body weight, but thirty pounds to me was some very real progress. I know it was mostly water as they tell you any time you start losing weight, but that was not important to me. I lost thirty pounds. I *lost THIRTY pounds*, not gained thirty but LOST it!

THAT TIME on the scale was life changing for me. The relief of seeing that scale go down for the first time in years, I realized, for once, something I was doing to change my lifestyle was finally working. I looked at that scale a few times. I looked to make sure the scaled wasn't touching the wall, I looked at the surroundings to make sure nothing was under the scale. I got on the scale two or three times, and it kept showing the exact same number. I remember there were people right there in the warehouse at the time. Everybody knew me at Suncor. For years I was known as Tony the big guy. All the people in the warehouse were very happy for me. They were giving me high fives. It was very cool. They all knew what was going on. Everybody was very happy for me, not that they could see a visible difference yet, but it was a moment to celebrate. From there it all snowballed, I kept at it and everybody started noticing, especially when I started to see huge losses by the Fall of 2016.

When I started losing weight, I was still doubting, understandably so because lots of people jump on the weight loss roller coaster; lose thirty pounds, then gain back fifty. Maybe you can relate if you've lost a bit and then suddenly you stop walking, you stop eating well, and then people see you with a chocolate bar in your hand again. It's tough to stick with a lifestyle change. People at work were right behind me as I kept at it. A little later as people were starting to notice it visibly they became even more encouraging.

It was a wonderful feeling; this was something I had

dreamed of for years. For about 14 years, not one day would go by that I did not wake up in the morning and wish that I was somebody else. Finally, I was becoming THAT somebody else. I had wished that I could lose weight. It was finally happening. It was unbelievable the happiness that this brought me. I was starting to be freed up in my mind. I was getting self confidence back, I was getting happiness back. The depression of being alone, of being this big was leaving my mind. I was finally getting hope back. That's why it's an important goal of this book to be giving hope, because I know how great it feels to finally get hope back.

Now I love walking. I walk every day, sometimes two or even occasionally three times a day. Now I just maintain my weight by walking. I initially walked to lose hundreds of pounds. I find a funny thing about walking is that for me now it's almost more of a mental benefit than physical. It clears my mind, it gets me going and I think about and process things. I get talking to myself quite a bit, not out loud, but in my head. Walking gets me thinking about where I'm going to go, or thinking about what's going on in my life, it just gets my mind rolling. It has a way of clearing my head.

When I'm at work in the oil patch, I work from 8:00 a.m. to 8:00 p.m. (or 8 p.m. to 8 a.m. on night shift). I would have to catch the bus at 6:50. I'll walk to the bus stop at 6:30. I would get up at 4:30 and go for a one-hour walk and be home at 5:30 to make breakfast and get ready for the day. I love it. If I miss a morning where I don't get up and go for a walk, I feel my whole day is ruined. Sometimes I get up and when I think about heading out for a walk as I roll over in bed, I smile, because I *can* actually walk. I am physically able to do this for four or five kilometres, no problem. Wow! A couple years ago this would've never happened. I would not have been able to do this.

It literally would have killed me! I could've had a heart

attack, or blown a lung walking 5 km. Now, even going through the airport, I'll take stairs instead of taking the escalator. I just zip up the stairs like it's nothing. I'm not out of breath, I'm not exhausted, I'm not dizzy, nothing! No problems. It's a very nice feeling. I look back and it's still like a dream, a beautiful, wide awake dream.

Building Momentum

I have seen in life the tendencies of the domino effect, or the butterfly effect. If one tiny change happens, if one little thing shifts, it can cause the whole world to be turned upside down. For me, those moments on the bus and on the airplane were that huge domino effect that set a course of events in place that brought on a massive chain reaction.

Taking the job at Suncor back in 2000 was one of those events. There were people I worked with who became friends, they initially challenged me and then later, they would help keep me on the straight and narrow. I did most of the dieting and walking just on my own, but they helped me along as well. Once I saw the weight starting to come off, and once things started getting a bit easier, then the process snowballed. It gained momentum and kind of took on a life of its own.

I went on holidays later in the summer of 2016 in August. I drove back to Newfoundland because I was still too big to fly. I wasn't going to take up two seats ever again if I could help it. I kept to my diet on the road, at my parents' home and all the way driving back to Alberta. My mom cooked healthy food for me while I was back home. I kept doing walks every day. I had little personal goals that I would set for myself. I had always wanted to have goals like that. I would set goals and reach them. I remember in September when I was back in Alberta I weighed myself. I had lost one hundred pounds using the exact same scale at work.

That was doing the unthinkable in August of 2016, I drove across the country on vacation, got spoiled by my mom for a week with down home cooking, drove back, eating in restaurants coming and going and *I still lost weight*. Straight away, anybody who has ever dieted would say, "You're going to put on weight, vacations and Mom's cooking are two of the biggest food downfalls known to man." As I just mentioned by September I had lost a hundred pounds. It can definitely be done. The impossible is possible.

I started to realize that years and years and years of always wanting to be somebody else, always wanting the weight to be off, it was actually happening. I was actually becoming that different guy; the new me. I've always wanted to not be handicapped anymore — especially this kind of handicap — the self-imposed disability. It was finally starting to happen, after years of dreaming about it. There was no turning back. Once clothes started fitting better, once I saw that change, there was no going back. Ever!

That's when the momentum of weight loss really kicked in. As the weight continued to come off, the walking got easier. Then seeing those results, down a hundred pounds, it became even easier to keep eating healthy. The results were all around me. Then not only had the exercises gotten easier, but the longer I went without processed sugar and the longer I went without junk food and pop, the easier it became to resist those cravings. Everything started getting easier.

I would get in the car one day, and notice, "Ha! This kind of fits a bit better", and I would slide the seat forward a little bit. Another day not long after that I noticed, "Hmmm...I don't have to wear my seatbelt extension." It seemed everyday there was something positive, a little victory to help build momentum.

I remember, one day I was at work and there was this forklift there that I could never fit in ever before. I just stepped up to it and got in it. Just like that! No trumpets playing, no fanfare, just another little victory. For the first year of weight loss, there were dozens, probably hundreds of all these little things that just started to happen, little things that I couldn't do for years that I was starting to be able to do again.

The Simple Formula

I stopped eating late at night. I was staying away from all the junk food. I was walking. I never even got a membership at a gym, not even exercising, I was only walking. It's like simple math. I started burning off more calories than I was taking in. I didn't need to count my points or my calories, I just walked and ate healthy.

That was it.

No diet pills, no stomach operation, no diet camps or spas, no instruction manuals, no online membership, no health club, no detox teas, no exercise program, no fees, no surcharges, nothing. I walked and ate healthy.

Simple Math — The part I understood, again not rocket science, but I knew that a 600-pound man needed to take in probably 6000 to 8000 calories a day just to maintain that type of weight. Suddenly I cut my calorie intake down to probably 1500/2000 calories a day or even less and then I started walking on top of that. Of course, the pounds were going to disappear! When you're overweight and you change your lifestyle as soon as you lose any number of pounds life becomes easier. It's like a snowball, when you're rolling that snowball down a hill it gets bigger and faster; momentum is on your side. This was what this was like for me, (except for me the snowball was getting smaller, not bigger). As the days went on and I stayed away from junk food, I was cutting out the sugar in my coffee to the point where I eventually took my coffee black or with only half a cream, little tweaks like that, things got even easier and the results continued to show up.

Areas of Progress

Every day, I kept noticing progress, maybe things that weren't a big deal to anyone else, but things that really, profoundly encouraged me. There was a statistical encouragement, watching the weight number fall, seeing and feeling the difference; that was neat. When I had finally dropped one hundred pounds that fall, I could put a pair of socks on again, I could finally fit into a pair of jeans again, I could finally start buying clothes again that weren't size 6 XL, but first it was a 5XL, then a 4XL …wow! I was getting smaller and all the numbers and clothes pointed in that direction.

Hitting Goals — I started the weight loss journey at 567 pounds in June of 2016. I desperately wanted to be at 399 pounds by New Years Day, 2017. On New Years Eve, 2016 I weighed myself and I was exactly 399 pounds. For the first time in over a decade, I was below the 400 mark. I wasn't 567 pounds. I wasn't four hundred and something pounds. I was finally "in the three zone" again. I was at 399. Then I felt I was really making serious progress. I was taking longer walks. I wasn't out of breath as much. I was starting to fit into my car easier. My clothes were getting looser. I could do up my jacket again for the first time in years. I could use the bathroom easier. I could wash myself in the shower easier. I could tie up my workbook boots now. I was having all these little gains, little wins almost every day!

Others Noticing, Positive Cycle — People were so happy for me making comments like, "Wow, you're really losing weight!"

Of course, I'd hear all the time, "Oh, I didn't recognize you."

I'd see people in the hallway that I hadn't seen in a month or two and I'd hear, "Holy - - - - Bussey! What happened to you. You're losing weight. This is great, keep it up."

I was doing all of this for myself. However, when others started to notice, it was like there was this built in encouragement that kept growing. Instead of being a downward spiral like when I had put the weight on (discouraged, feel lousy, eat, feel worse, eat more, discouraged more…) now there was an upward spiral of events: eat healthy, walk, feel great, people encourage me, I feel great, keep eating healthy, keep walking, keep feeling even better… this cycle was and still is a wonderful thing!

Back to the Bus — I had a thought one day that pretty much stopped me in my tracks. I thought, "I'm going to start taking the bus. I would fit into a seat now, no problem."

So, I parked my car, and I got on the bus. I went to the back seat of the bus. It had been years since I'd taken the bus from town to work. I got on the bus. I pulled the seatbelt across my waist and, "click." It FIT! Wow. I left the car at home, and I've been taking the bus to work regularly ever since that day. I take the bus *every* day now. As I said, often it will be two or three weeks before I need to fill my car with gas. I used to need two or three fill ups a week when I was driving back and forth to work. Do you see what's happening here? My weight loss has been so huge it's even been good for the environment!

I remember one day I got on the bus, when I was in the mid-300's weight range and the bus was fairly packed. I found a seat. As the bus filled up, before, nobody would sit next to me. However, this gentleman came down the aisle. There were a few other empty seats here and there that he could have chosen, but this guy came along and he chose to sit next to me. I'll never forget it. I realized that I wasn't that big huge guy that nobody wanted to or couldn't sit next to. I was beside the empty seat that he picked over other vacant spots, he chose to come and sit next to me. With the armrest down he still had room to sit comfortably with his seat belt on. I couldn't wipe the smile off my face for hours that day I'm sure.

That simple little bus story, in my mind was one of the highlights of the whole lifestyle change story. You see, right at that very moment, I was "normal." Most people strive to be extraordinary, to stand out from the crowd, to be noticed, to be the centre of attention. If I can refresh your memory, an obese person strives to be one of thousands, to fit in, not to be noticed or stand out anymore. When I finally became *that* guy, "I'm just normal, one in a crowd of many. I go to work, I'm not singled out or stared at anymore."

When that guy came down the centre aisle of the bus and sat next to me, that's when I wanted to let out a massive, "YESSSS! Finally! I'm here." …and start fist pumping and giving high-fives up and down the centre aisle. I refrained and stayed cool though, but I'm pretty sure a smile leaked out onto my face right away.

I kept losing weight and losing more weight, to the weight I'm at now, 230 pounds. I will never forget that bus ride. Now, I get on a plane when I travel longer distances. I can. I fit. When I get on a plane, I'm just one of hundreds of regular passengers who fits in an airplane seat. No special seatbelt extension. Nobody knows anything. I'm not singled out. I'm just inconspicuous. People might not even just glance at me, or even notice me at all, not even a little bit because I'm just one of hundreds of normal people. It feels so wonderful to be an average Joe again, a regular guy.

On a funny note, it's still habit for me to go to the back of the bus, to look for a seat for more room. Old habits die hard I guess!

Rental Cars and Other Rides — I feel like I can go anywhere in the world now just because I can *fit* in an airplane seat. The limitations are also gone because when I get wherever I'm flying, I can fit into a rental car. I don't have to stay at the airport or just walk everywhere.

At the airport in Victoria, BC before I changed my lifestyle I was picking up a rental vehicle. I asked the lady at the counter, "What's the biggest vehicle that you have here?"

She said, "Well, how many people do you have?" I guess she didn't notice she was talking to a 600-pound man.

I said, "You're not understanding the question," and she laughed.

She awkwardly responded, "Oh!" She looked at me, and she was a sweetheart about it. She gave me this big handful of keys and continued, "Go out in the parking lot and try them out and see whatever fits. Come back and we'll set you up."

I went out into the parking lot. I walked around, and I found this huge Chevy Suburban, I think it was, a seven passenger Suburban. I said, "Well, if that huge thing doesn't fit then I'm in trougle. We'll have to *walk* all the way to Victoria." I got into that massive Suburban and I could barely fit in that thing. The vehicle was huge, but behind that steering wheel even when I put the seat all the way back and I put the seat as low as it would go, I tilted the steering wheel all the way up it was still tight in there. Then I got in my head in but it was still stuck up into the ceiling. I could just barely fit in that huge beast, but I got it, and that's what Emma and I used to see Victoria. Driving around Victoria in a huge seven passenger Suburban, as a 600-pound dude, you're attracting some serious staring with that.

These days, I can show up to an airport car rental desk and they can offer me a little Smart Car, I'll take it. It doesn't bother me. There's no stress for me. I can fit in any rental car. I don't have that anxiety about rental cars anymore because I'm just a normal person. I blend into the airport crowd, I'm one of thousands of normal people. Nobody takes a second look at me, nobody stares at me, I'm just another face in the crowd.

When I go up to the counter, and ask what they have to rent it doesn't matter what their answer is, I'm ready with my standard answer, "Perfect, give it to me."

I feel that God gave me the guys I've gotten to know at work, a group that is like family. My blood relatives, my real family members are on the east coast. My daughter in Red Deer, is 600 km away, but those guys from work are like a close-knit family. On each shift there's 34 of us right there in the tire shop and they are the best group of guys, funny, charming, hard working. The strength and encouragement I have received from them through this process, has been great. They're always rooting for me. They were so happy for me when I lost the weight. They are a wonderful group of guys.

In the heavier days, if one of those guys from work dropped by and came to pick me up and said, "Come on Bussey, let's go for a coffee," it would break my heart because getting in the car to hang out with them was a huge issue. Will I fit in the car, will this be possible? I didn't want to by anti-social with my family. Now, that I've lost the weight, a buddy might call me up to connect and it's no problem to do it. I can fit now. Let's go! Before, I didn't go out very often because I hated the awkward process of going out with people. There was a lot of tension around all of the issues that could go wrong, just because I was huge; vehicle size, bathroom options, temperature, mobility, walking distance, fatigue, stamina, booth or table, strong enough chairs — there were dozens of things that could complicate the outing with Big Tony on the scene.

If I got tired early during an outing and I couldn't walk back, could I call a cab, would I be able to get one large enough? Now I could. If I got sick today I could go to a hospital and not have to worry about if I'm going to fit on a stretcher, or fit in a hospital bed or room, or use their bathroom facilities, or if they're going to be able to check my blood pressure.

Hair Cut — In the "Big Tony" days it was difficult to get my hair cut. I've been going to the same barber for about 16 years. I still go to the same barber today. He used to see me at my biggest and now he has seen me lose the weight. I went to his shop one day back when I was heavy. I used to hate getting my hair cut because I couldn't fit in his chair. One day, and I sat in the chair, and that little silver bar that's below the chair, that metal bar you put your feet on, I destroyed it. Being uncomfortable in that tight chair, I tried to adjust myself, but here I was pushing with my feet on this bar that couldn't handle my weight.

I was sitting in the chair and I had my feet down there, and I pushed down to adjust myself. I pushed that silver bar right down to the floor and the bar just stayed at the floor level. I broke his chair. He was always a wonderful guy, he still is. He didn't say anything. He just looked at me but he didn't say a word. He cut my hair. Even to pump up the chair, to lift me up a bit, he couldn't pump me up an inch because I was too heavy. He cut my hair. It would usually be three or four months between appointments, because I hated going through that process, I couldn't stand it. When I went back the next time, he had all new chairs.

I continue to go to that same guy all the time. He's always amazing. We'll sit and talk, because he remembers me very well, and he'll tell his friends about this customer, "This guy was huge." Now I go in there and I get into the chair and if feels great. I fit in the chair, he can jack me up, he can swivel me around in the chair and cut my hair, it's great. I always leave him a nice tip, because I feel bad about breaking his chair years ago. I figured if I keep going there for the next twenty years the tips will eventually pay for the chairs that I broke.

Normal Tony — If I go into a mall, if I go into a box store, I'm just one of the people. Before, I was always the huge guy, "Oh, there's the big guy. That's big T. That's 'big Tony' they call him. He's certainly a big man!" I might have been the biggest person in Fort McMurray! I can't imagine anybody being bigger than I was.

This Thing Has a Back Seat? — Every time I would get into my car, I'd feel a little bit more room. I remember for years I could never fit in the backseat of my car. When I had lost quite a bit of weight, I remember one day I brought my car home. I parked it and I thought, for whatever crazy reason, "I'm going to try to get in the back seat." I was at the parkade in my condo. I got in the back seat of my car and I just sat there. I had the biggest grin on my face, because I was sitting there in the backseat of my car. "Nice. I have NEVER been in the backseat of this car. Cool." I can't imagine how that looked on the security cameras. Is this guy robbing this car? No, he's just climbing in the back seat. Cleaning? Nope. Looking for something? Nope. Up to something suspicious? Doesn't look like it. He's just sitting there. Wait. He's smiling. It's a really big smile. Is he drunk? Probably.

Confession time: To this day, I'll go to the parking garage sometimes and I'll sit in the back seat of my car. Just for fun. Just to sit there. Awkward.

Cab Just for Fun — One time in Calgary, I didn't want to drive downtown, I left my car at the hotel. Half the reason I did it was not so much the drive downtown. That was just kind of an excuse. The real reason I left the car at the hotel was just so that I could call a cab. I couldn't fit in most of them before. If I did have to get a cab in extreme circumstances, I'd have to make sure it was a minivan so I could get in the backseat. I remember the cab that showed up in Calgary was a tiny little car. I got in the front seat, and I fit with ease. I'm sure the cab driver must have seen me smiling the whole trip downtown and he was thinking exhaust was leaking into the backseat and killing brain cells.

Better Health — I also remember when I started to

notice that my skin was clearing up. I wasn't getting the cuts on my forehead anymore. My eye wasn't fogging over, it wasn't glazing over anymore. I wasn't getting the tingling in my legs anymore. I wasn't waking up in the middle of the night choking anymore. All of those health benefits were great, most of them because the sugar and deep-fried foods were out of my life. The cravings for junk food were gone. I didn't crave that anymore. I had lots more energy; tons of it. I had the energy I have now, and beyond.

One day I even ran for the first time since I was probably a teenager. I tried running. I still can't run a lot because of the twenty to thirty pounds of loose skin that I'm carrying, but I ran. That was kind of cool.

I'm not out of breath these days. I now know I can climb up two hundred stairs. I did that in Edmonton. I went for a walk while I was there, and there are these stairs that went up from the park that's in the valley and when you take the stairs all the way up, you're right downtown. I think it's about two hundred stairs. I got to the top of those steps and I just kept walking. At the airport now or in the mall, whenever I can, I don't hesitate to take the stairs. I don't take the escalator. I love taking the stairs. Just because I can!

Keep on Walking — As I became *Tony the Normal* I lost my anxiety about the danger of driving on the roads or slipping and falling on the sidewalks and I became a committed walker, not afraid of a spill. When I started losing weight I wouldn't stop my walks even in the rain, the snow or the intense heat.

In August of 2016, I visited Peterborough, Ontario. It was three months after I started losing my weight. I had lost about seventy pounds at that time. It was very hot there; forty degrees with the humidity, and I still went out for my daily walk then. Sweat was pouring off me but I kept at it. I was pretty resilient for a big guy. I tried not to make excuses, I just kept pressing through, trying to make the best of it.

Clothes Shopping - I had mentioned earlier the George Richards Big and Tall store where I would shop when I visited Emma down in Red Deer. I went back a couple years ago, when I started losing the weight and I had almost lost all of my weight. I went in there one day to do some shopping. I looked around for a while and finally a sales lady said to me that they didn't have clothes here small enough for me. That sales lady knew me from years of visiting. She had come to know me as a regular client. As I visited there she would see me and my gradual weight gain over those years and then my gradual weight loss that came with the lifestyle change. She said, "Honey, you don't have to come back here anymore! I'll miss you, but you don't ever want to come back here."

Wow! That felt good. So. Good. I felt like crying. It was joyful. I can't describe to you the sense of relief that washed over me with those words. Relief! If there's anything I feel through all of this, it's relief. Every day I feel that deep sense of relief.

If I can, let me explain this feeling a bit more. Nowadays I can wake up in the morning and just be a normal person. Almost everybody has a desire, maybe a secret ambition to be something they want to be, to do something big in the world and be the best that they can be. As a big guy that size, I've already told you that my dream was simply to fit in and not be noticed at all; to no longer stick out like a sore thumb; to *not* be stared at. When that sales lady said to me that the store didn't have clothes small enough, it was like Christmas! It was the best news! It finally hit me, "I'm just a normal, regular guy now. I can shop at normal stores!" I had my life back.

The feeling of relief and joy is overwhelming. Finally, after fourteen years of extreme heaviness and more than twenty years being overweight I was normal! I felt relieved because to struggle with that huge weight, that amount of weight, for years and years and to go through all of that negative emotion, disappointment and discouragement and to live every day feeling lousy, it was too much to carry. I just wanted to be somebody else, to finally be done with all of that darkness, done with all the burden of constant *heavy* emotion. It's almost indescribable to put into words what I felt when I heard her tell me that I wouldn't ever have to come back to the Big and Tall store. I was like Edmund Hillary getting to the top of Mount Everest, or how Columbus must have felt when he reached the new world. When I reached that pinnacle, achieved my goal it was like, "Wow! I finally got here. I made it. I've finally made it." It's still amazing to me. Every. Single. Day. I still feel that sense of overwhelming relief.

The Day Socks Returned — I can't remember exactly what day it was, if it was after I lost that first hundred pounds or a bit before that, but I still had not been wearing socks. I hadn't tried to put socks on for quite some time, so I thought I would try it this one particular day. I tried to put them on and lo and behold, I could actually get them on.

In many ways, the socks have been very symbolic for me. The lack of socks represented pain, discomfort, social awkwardness, embarrassment and shame. When I could start wearing socks again it seemed like life was really coming together for me. It had been three years of not being able to wear socks which symbolizes to me the worst part of the worst season of my life. Thank God that season is over.

Right now, today, writing this book, I'm still glowing from putting my on socks four hours ago! Seriously. I have socks, beyond socks, beyond socks in my drawer at home now. It's over the top. I'm a sock-o-holic. To be able get up in the morning, get ready for the day, to put the socks on, to put jeans on, to put a shirt on, clothes that are decent clothes, it's nothing short of incredible for me. Those socks symbolize everything bad turning to good. It symbolizes being normal. It symbolizes fitting in. It symbolizes not being in pain. It symbolizes that I don't smell bad or have chafing or rashes. It symbolizes that this weight problem is kicked. It's done. That old life is over and done. I still have to pinch myself. It's over. There's no more of that. I have a brand-new lifestyle. I'm free.

It lasted for about three years, the season without socks. The first day I could put socks on was a great day in my life. Why would I ever choose even a taste of junk food compared to that victory? I don't want it. People ask me if I'll ever go back to the old life again, eating even a little bit of junk and I have to say, "Never again". Why? Because I can wear socks now. I'm wearing socks right now as this is being written. Isn't this exciting? If I could summarize everything wonderful that has happened to me in the last two and half years, sum it up in just one word, that's easy: "socks".

Shoes and Boots — I had been going through more shoes because of how they smelled but also, I was walking funny and ruining my footwear quickly. I look at my feet now still surprised that I didn't have more problems with my feet. Again, thanks for the prayers Mom!

Tying up my boots at work is a big joke now. The boys at work, sometimes they'll laugh at me because my boots will be tied up and I'll bend over and I'll tighten them up even further, just because I can! I could never do that before. Who knew it would be such a luxury to have nice tight work boots on your feet?

Another thing this brings up is the socks, they serve as a vapour barrier to absorb any perspiration from your feet. A fresh pair of socks every day keep your footwear from become damp and keeps them clean and fresh. Not wearing socks makes your shoes or boots smell awful. The accompanying smell from not wearing socks is no longer a problem in my life. The social stigma of having stinky feet is gone. I can visit people now in their homes, because as we know, Canadians take their shoes off when they go into some one's home. It's polite eh?

Family Visits — I mentioned earlier that I couldn't visit Emma's family in Red Deer because of my stinky feet, especially Penny's one sister, her name is Sonya. She was always insisting that I come in and visit. I always declined. I would always leave the wrong impression that I didn't want to be with them, that perhaps I had something against them. Why doesn't Tony come in to see us? Does he not like us? What's the problem?

A year ago, I was visiting Red Deer and I stopped in and saw Sonya. I went on in and we were sitting there talking and I told her the story. I said, "Sonya, do you know the real reason I didn't come in?"

She said, "what's that?"

I told her that. She cried.

It felt great; not that I enjoy making ladies cry, it just felt great to finally have the truth out in the open, not the awkward story that I didn't want to come hang out, that there seemed to be some kind of problem. For years I had wanted to tell her the truth about having stinky feet, but I was too ashamed, too embarrassed. I felt bad about my foot odour problem, but it felt great to get rid of that social barrier. It felt amazing. I knew, they're the type of family that if I would have told them the truth, they would have still said, "Come on in. Who cares? We'll put up with the stink. We love you."

I Had Forgotten About Shorts — I bought my first shorts for the first time in about 25 years when I went to Mexico this year. I also wore my first pair of sandals. The last couple summers, I was still be going out for walks, dressed in my usual heavy clothes that looked more like a tent than clothes. Even if it was over 30 degrees Celsius the only difference in my attire was having a t-shirt on, going for a walk in sweltering heat with long pants. I just never thought about wearing shorts thinking I needed to keep my shameful body fat covered up, even after the fat was gone. Then in Mexico I wore shorts. It was shocking how cool and refreshing it was. I'll never wear jeans again next summer! This is great. I felt like a kid again! It's a lot less hot than wearing long pants. Who knew? Apparently most of the population knew, I had just forgotten about shorts.

I had to go buy all new clothes. What a terrible problem to have! Because I was spending $500/month more on junk food and eating out and now I might spend $500/month less on gas, I've freed up some budget to spend on clothes.

I wasn't smart in the beginning because I bought nice, new clothes when I started losing weight. Then I'd lose more weight and just like that I'd realize, "These clothes are too big for me now!" I'd have to head down to the Salvation Army donation centre saying, "I've got a brand new hundred-dollar pair of jeans here for ya', only been worn twice!"

I'm thankful for everything I have, more than ever. I don't feel that I'm arrogant or materialistic about it, it's just that I take pride in things now, like my clothes. I fold my underwear and I put them in a dresser. I fold my jeans and I fold up my socks. Before, my entire wardrobe was horrible, everything was stained, dirty and abused. It was not nice.

I didn't have the ability to eat a dozen Timbits and juggle a Double Big Mac and a Diet Pepsi all at the same time without spilling it all over my clothes on a regular basis — I don't have that ability to balance food when my arms probably weighed 80 pounds each and my fingers were the size of sausages. I'd wash those clothes and throw them in the dryer and then I'd just leave it all in the dryer, taking it out as I needed it. I only had three pairs of gym pants and several stained shirts. I just had very little self-respect.

These days, I've got all kinds of nice clothes. I fold everything. I take more pride in the things that I have because I have more pride in myself. When you don't care about yourself, you don't care about the things that you have.

Furniture — About one year into the weight loss journey, my first big purchase was a brand new bed set. My couch was ruined. After having a 600-pound lazy guy watching hundreds of movies and eating tons of junk food on it, that banana couch had structurally bent to its max! It finally retired, broken, warped and bruised. When I had first moved into my condo, I rented the condo off a friend of mine. I bought all of his furniture and it was pretty good quality - not the quality to withstand my big weight - but great furniture. After sitting on that couch for a few months I had warped it and eventually bent it out of shape. I got rid of the old couch and I bed and it was a very happy moment, one of those moments where I couldn't wipe the smile off my face for days. I am now the proud owner of a non-banana couch.

It was always a dream of mine to have this really nice comfortable bed. I bought a queen size bed frame, I actually had a frame that wouldn't break, I was so pleased about that. I bought a nice mattress and a box spring too. I don't take them for granted because every single thing I own feels like a gift from God. As a result, I take way better care of my possessions. There's not a morning now where I don't get up and make my bed. It's the first thing I do before I even have my coffee.

Bathrooms — This might not sound like a big deal, but I can go to the bathroom any time, any place and not be limited by the size of the bathroom stall, or not be restricted in what I eat at work because I can have a bathroom break and not destroy my life to do it. I can eat normal meals at work now. I can use any bathroom anywhere. It's incredibly liberating.

Movies - I remember when I first lost the weight and Emma could sit closer to me in a movie theatre, it felt really amazing. I said to her, "Emma, you can sit next to me now." Once again, I must have had a smile on my face for days.

Remember, she's a grown woman today and she can sit right next to me. When she was little, she could not sit next to me because I was too big. Now, we sit in a movie theatre and I can put the armrest down. She can put her pop or snacks in the cupholder.

Massage — I went for my first massage a couple weeks ago. My work has a benefits package where I can get a massage and they cover most of the cost. I could never take advantage of that benefit before, because I always thought it would be senseless to try to massage through all that fat. I didn't want to be on the table, and just being massive, undressed. It sounded like a recipe for embarrassment. What had I been missing? It was wonderful to have a massage. It felt great.

Making Plans — Now I've got all kinds of plans. I love going out for walks and I plan to do that every day for the rest of my life. I realize now that Fort McMurray has many beautiful walking trails to enjoy that I didn't know about before. I couldn't go out for walks before. Now if somebody invites me out, I'll go anywhere, no problem. I can go to a movie theatre, no problem. I can sit down at any restaurant, table or booth. Whatever! No issues.

I'll go for a walk down to the mall and see if there's anyone I know there to go and talk to. Before, I couldn't do that. I've become more social again. That's who I was the whole time, but I was kind of trapped inside that huge body.

Holidays — Emma and I have a Christmas get-together, either I'll go down to Red Deer right before Christmas or just after Christmas, and we'll have our own little time; a gift exchange and just be together. I'll give Penny, her mom, some money to buy some gifts for Christmas Day when I'm not there, and every year I ask Emma, "what did I buy you this year?" I don't even have a clue.

When we connect at Christmas, because my birthday's on January the ninth, we'll have a little Christmas *and* birthday event together. I'll take her out for a nice dinner to The Keg Steakhouse or something nice like that. I'll give her a gift just from me, and she'll give me something and we'll have our little date together. It's all very nice.

I haven't been home to Newfoundland for Christmas since 1999. So, I'm thinking maybe next year, 2019, I might go home, have a Christmas back on the Rock. Mom and Dad are getting older and Mom really wants me to come home one year for Christmas. The worst thing with traveling up there in the wintertime is the weather and I might end up get stuck up there; literally snowed in, airports closed, highways closed, it's not uncommon. That's a big reason why in other years, having to drive home wasn't possible. Flying was not an option for the big Tony, so getting home just wasn't realistic. When you're driving across Canada in the wintertime, anything can happen. Now that I can fly, it's a different story.

Travel — Last summer, I took Emma home for first time to Newfoundland with me and she finally met my parents. For years, I couldn't take her to Newfoundland to meet my own family. Here she is, the dearest person in my life and I couldn't even introduce her to my parents! She was 17-years old before she met my mom and dad.

Emma and I rented a car back home after flying into St. John's, the first time I had driven across Newfoundland in probably twenty years. She doesn't like driving. She gets a bit sick if she's in the car too long. From St.John's I drove as far west as Deer Lake. We got a hotel there for the night, then the next day we drove up the Northern Peninsula to my home town. Of course, Mom and Dad took right to her. As soon as we went into the house, mom came over to her and loved on her. I thought she was going to cry. She gave Emma a big hug. My dad gave her a big hug. It was a lot for Emma to take in because they're all basically strangers to her. Now she's finally met them.

Driving up the coast, is as gorgeous a drive as you'd ever see. On the one side, there are the Gros Morne Mountains, on the other side it's beautiful forests, hills and ocean. Someday I'd like to visit Gros Morne National Park, and enjoy the beauty, take the boat and go right into the fjords, and then climb up Gros Morne. I can't wait to do it. Every other time that I've been home, it's only been for about a week; not really enough time to go hiking. Now that I can fly home, I'll have the time.

Now I can. In so many ways I can do anything; I am actually able to do things that used to be impossible. It's wonderful; I'm free to do so much that I could literally not do before. I want to do it all, but I want to do it all right away. Every day, I'm thinking, "I want to do this, I want to do that," because now I can! There's nothing stopping me now.

I got to speak down in Calgary this past May, a public speaking engagement that I enjoyed a lot. I showed them my big fat pants. That was kind of cool. When you show them that, that's when you get the "wow" factor, because they're huge. I feel like I'm holding up a circus tent from the Ringling Brothers, there is enough material there for three pairs of jeans. You could blanket a twin bed with the amount of denim in them. It's not only that I can do things I've always dreamed of doing, I'm doing things I never even dreamed of doing. I never thought in a million years I'd be invited to Calgary to share my story in front of a crowd and show off my sixty-six-inch waist on my jeans that were too small for me. How crazy is that? What obese person would even think of that possibility? I sure didn't.

Emma Involved — When Emma and I flew into St John's, Newfoundland, she was able to meet my cousin for the first time. We stayed in St. John's a couple nights and did an interview with CBC Newfoundland. Not only did Emma meet my folks, she met extended family. She met cousins. She met friends. She saw where I grew up. She saw where I lived. She saw all the little things that I used to tell her about, experiences I had as a child. Now I could finally show her those very spots and she loved it. We'd get up in the morning, she'd ask, "Who are we going to go visit today, dad?" She loved that part.

Emma is a young woman and it's a delight to be fully involved in her life now with no weight restrictions. In a few years, she might have kids of her own. I hope to do with those kids what I wish I could have done with Emma.

Today, Emma is probably the proudest of anybody at what I've done, losing 337 pounds. Her mother has told me that Emma is proud. I've heard Emma say it herself, that she's proud of me!

Emma was involved with me in the CBC interview back in Newfoundland. She was a bit nervous, but I talked to her before. I said, "Well, Emma, you're going to be on the internet now. Once you're out there, you're there for good." I'm sure that made her even more nervous, but I made sure she was comfortable with it. She was like an old pro. doing the interview. She totally nailed it.

Emma said something remarkable in that interview we did for the CBC that really meant a lot to me. She said, "Before this, my dad only *observed* my life. Now he can *be a part* of my life, *involved* in my life."

That was very true. Before when I was *Tony the Large*, "we" would do things together, but she'd be the only one really *doing* it. I'd only be *observing* it. Now, we can actually **DO** things together. Before, I'd go pick her up in the car and all it would be was dinner and a movie. Now we can go and do anything! We can travel places and we can really do things together. Sometimes we go to a mall to look around. We can do that, we can walk together. I plan on taking her on trips. Three years ago, I didn't want to go anywhere or do anything, because I didn't want to be seen anywhere in public. Now, I'll go anywhere she wants.

Pictures — Now, I'm all about uploading selfies on my phone. If you see my Facebook profile, you'll find a few shots of me before the weight loss, but not many. As I said, I *hated* having my picture taken. Now on my Facebook, there are dozens of selfies. I'm not very vain or full of myself, but it's certainly nice to not feel embarrassed of my photos. I feel like I'm a normal person. Of course I want to smile for the camera now because I had missed that for fourteen years!

Levelling Off — Right now, my weight's floating around 230 - 232 pounds (not kilos). Once I get skin surgery, I'll be down around 210, maybe even 205. That's where I want to stay. I don't want to get any smaller than that. People keep telling me, "Don't lose anymore weight. You're going to start to look sick." Which is kind of weird because three years ago, everybody was telling me, "You've got to lose some weight or you'll be sick…or dead." Now that the comments are "don't lose any more weight," I find I just can't keep anybody happy.

Noticeable Heart Change

Less Angry - I've had a lot of road rage in the past. I'd be driving alone and a guy might not put on his signal, or somebody would cut me off and I would be livid. It would make me red with rage. Now, things that I'm like, "pff." I don't care now. It doesn't get to me. Before, it wouldn't take much to set me off. Now everybody even comments about how I'm so laid back these days. There's just nothing to be mad about anymore. I don't know. I guess that when you're going around with life, with 330 pounds on your back, the pain on your feet, rashes on your stomach, you know, loneliness, uncertainty; everything else used to seem magnified, more intense. Now it's relaxed.

Positivity — I have literally been healing from the inside out. I have been becoming less handicapped, gradually. Losing all the excess weight, there was an emotional weight that lifted too, a healing that was coming with it. The dream of being normal again was happening. I was getting my life back. As I lost the weight, I gained happiness, I was gaining my emotional strength again. Eventually, I was becoming my old self again. Problems and opposition were not making me as upset anymore. I was gradually becoming more relaxed, I was happier about life, I was more optimistic every day. It was much easier to have a positive outlook. It felt like as the bad effects and attitudes would leave, as they'd go out the door, the door stayed open and all this good stuff started coming in.

New Found Joy — As I mentioned earlier, for me, there are few things that compare to the simple joy of buying normal clothes after being so limited in my choices for fourteen years; a variety of nice new clothes in a regular size, off a regular rack at normal store at a normal price. Might I suggest something: you will never find happiness at the bottom of a bag of chips that you're meant to find from feeling good about yourself. Or for that matter, at the bottom of a beer bottle or at the tip of a syringe.

I'm not trying to be conceited at all, but just looking in the mirror brings me great joy, having the ability to put on a normal shirt sized *men's large*, wearing normal clothes purchased at a common store, not a big and tall specialty clothing store, just to be a normal person and not have to look at a huge blob in the mirror, it's AWESOME. I'm proud of myself. Again, not in an arrogant way, but I'm really proud of myself, by God's grace, with the help of my mom's prayers, I'm changed. I got up this morning I shaved, I brushed my teeth. Then I got to put on a nice pair of jeans, I was able to put on socks and not fall over, I put on a nice fresh shirt. I looked in the mirror and saw a normal guy, I was getting all gushy. I was very proud of myself.

It was even better than chocolate chip cookie dough ice-cream. It was better than a Nanaimo bar (google it non-Canadians). That food *rush* is temporary, short-term dust-in-the-wind kind of stuff, but this joy is permanent. Getting dressed every morning and just having normal clothes is like a permanent tub of cookie dough ice-cream. This smile on my face now about wearing socks is like a never-ending Nanaimo bar. No matter what I'm doing these days, no matter how bad of a day, no matter what happens, having lost this weight, I don't have to deal with that pain and all the negative stuff anymore. I can't really put that into words, but that's why I had to write the chapter about what it's like being obese. That was hard to talk about all those details, to write it down. Contrast is a great teacher. Only when you understand how awful, extreme, painful, lonely and frustrated my life was can you appreciate how much more joyful and wonderful life is now!

That pain was years in the making, but the change happened in an instant! Done. Boom. Just like that. I can't really explain it. Something just switched, something changed in my mindset. It was almost like a cover came off, or a cork popped. It's like something showed up, like a strength stored up in my mind finally revealed itself. It was like my whole attitude changed. In an instant, everything changed to where I became fully aware of how vulnerable I was. I instantly became sure of what I had to do. I became totally aware of how beautiful life is and that I was passing it up for junk food.

Here I am, a Canadian male, living in a country where three quarters of the world would die to have a chance to live here. I have a wonderful job that a lot of Canadians would love to have. I have a smart, sweet, beautiful daughter, I have great friends. I have the ability and the freedom to go and do whatever I want whenever I want and the only thing stopping me, the only thing holding me back was me. I was putting myself in a self-made prison. There was a whole wonderful life out there that I couldn't access because of all the weight that was on my frame.

Now that's gone.

For fourteen years increasing from 400 to almost 600 pounds, I realized the world was not designed for me, it was not equipped to deal with my huge body. I couldn't access much of life, I couldn't do things. It was the weight, that excess fat that held me back. Now, like I have said many times I'm free! It was like I chose to amputate a vital part of me.

Seeing the seats on the evacuation plane and the bus, that was my get-out-of-jail-free card! For whatever reason that was the positive kick in the butt that I needed. It was free. No gym membership, no pills to buy, no stomach surgery to have, no eating plan to follow and products to purchase, it was free, but it cost me dearly, I cost me everything! I had to give up all my best friends. That bag of chips, I would have married those chips if it was legal. The ice cream, the donuts, I had to give up the comfort of every one of those dear "friends."

If I can recap the old season this way: When I got up in the morning, I had the tingly feeling in my legs, the skin on my forehead changed to a darker colour, I had dark circles under my eyes and the one eye was blurry and emitting a discharge. I was getting chest pains and my feet were killing me. I was getting bloody rashes on my belly and between my thighs. I was waking up in the middle of the night choking, unable to breathe. I could barely walk to the car without getting out of breath. My body was sending me signals. I knew what was happening. I was becoming very aware that I definitely wouldn't reach the age of 45. I was 41 when it all changed. I really don't think I would have seen 43. That would have devastated my daughter. What a waste, what a waste of a life! I didn't want to die. I knew if I died I'd die alone. I've already mentioned how I'd turn in for the night, not knowing if I was going to wake up. Whenever I went out somewhere, I didn't know if I was going to have a heart attack.

If I didn't keep at it, if I didn't struggle through the withdrawals from the sugar and diet soda, if I didn't struggle through the pain of walking, to start losing weight what would have happened? If I didn't fight through and just give everything up cold turkey, would I have gotten another chance?

I'm very thankful I took the first steps and kept going until I reached this new happy life. It was worth the sacrifice and the continued effort to stay here. My life no longer sucks. It's amazing now. Can you read it? Can you hear my smile?

8

Lifestyle Change

To say my life has changed is an understatement if there ever was one. Not only has my life changed, but many areas of my lifestyle have changed *significantly* and *dramatically*.

I have kept some physical memories of those heavy days, just a few things. I have a pair of jeans size 66-inches which were getting tight, one shirt, a belt and one jacket. At work, I have kept an old 7XL winter jacket that the supervisor had specially brought in for me and I've got an old pair of work overalls size 8XLT. I currently weigh 230 pounds and I have been consistently at this weight for over six months. I believe this to be my permanent weight. I hope to have the excess skin removed in the near future. Eventually I want to get to the point where I'll have lost the weight for so long that nobody will believe I was ever that big if it weren't for the physical proof.

My lifestyle is entirely different now. I'd like to get down to the nitty gritty on "how" my lifestyle changed.

BY TONY BUSSEY & WITH MARK GRIFFIN

We're NOT Dogs, We Don't Need a Treat

I really like this line "We're not dogs, we don't need a treat." Since I started to change my lifestyle I've really latched onto this idea. We truly don't need a treat every now and then to keep us going or to reward ourselves.

Food has always been a type of reward for me ever since I was a young boy growing up in Newfoundland. In a small town, food was a very big part of the culture and food, even for little kids, was a reward. It's something happy, it's something good, no matter if you're well off or if you're poor, it made no difference. If your mother could bake you were doing great. She would say, "You did a good job with your chores! Good boy. Here's a cookie!" With that, everything was right in the world.

Every home would have cookies. Everybody would enjoy a treat together. There'd be lots of popping by a friends house or family home, hanging out in the kitchen, having a cup of tea and a snack. Down east it's a part of the culture for friends and family to visit anytime, even at 9:30 p.m. expecting to sit down to a five-course meal where three courses of that are cookies, pies and sweets! It's only right to offer it to people who are kind enough to drop in and visit with you in your home on a miserable snowy or rainy night. If you don't eat what's offered, then the hosts would be insulted. There was no real emphasis on health. Food just made everyone feel happy so it was served and gladly eaten.

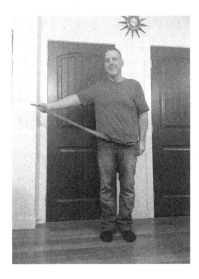

My old belt.

EVEN TO THIS day that reward mentality, that treat thinking is in my mind. I'll be a bit of a hypocrite. I won't eat junk food myself, but I'll go and buy some junk food for somebody else because I'll know it might make them happy. After all, it used to bring me a smile, so I try to bring them a smile. I'll get them a chocolate bar or an ice cream to brighten their day. I think when I bring a snack or a food treat as a gift, what I intend to bring is *happiness in a wrapper*. That's an instilled mentality for me.

No matter what was going on in my life, I always treated food as an escape to a happy place. If something good was happening, food was a part of the celebration. If something bad was happening, food was a comforting escape to feel better for a moment. Food seemed to be the answer for everything.

As an escape, a treat or a reward, food was slowly killing me, especially when I was at my heaviest. If the day was extra painful, or the day at work was extra long, food was something to look forward to at the end of the day. I often felt like I had nothing else to look forward to. If I knew I was going home and I had a big bag of chips in the cupboard, or if I had my favourite ice cream in the fridge it was something to get me through the day. It kept me going. However, we aren't driven just by our basic animal instincts, we are a step up in the animal kingdom. *We're not dogs, we don't need treats.*

I recognize that I've continued using food as a reward my entire life. I can eat the healthier "treats" I eat now until the day I die. I'm not a dog who eats likes there might not ever be another meal. I can control my cravings.

I don't eat excessively. I eat eggs, but I might have bacon once every couple of weeks. I eat meats, I eat veggies. I call it an old Newfoundland diet, except I don't touch bread. Mostly I eat meat and veggies. Unlike the old Newfie diet I also stay away from potatoes, I don't have them very often, especially Fries or anything deep-fried.

As a good Newfie, I eat seafood; salmon, codfish, shellfish, even a bit of shrimp, I love my seafood roots. I really enjoy a piece of salmon with some broccoli and some cauliflower or other veggies. It's delicious. I remember when I first started eating healthy and I went home that summer of 2016, my mom was cooking healthy for me. She was so sick of broccoli and cauliflower by the time I left I think I made her sick of it. Poor mother.

Food As Fuel — I've had to learn that I can no longer look at food as my reward at the end of the day. That is significant for me. I had to begin to look at food as *fuel* — the energy source that makes my body function. I heard this once, the analogy of a car and food. If you were told at the beginning of your life that you were going to get one vehicle and that's the only vehicle you're going to have the rest of your life, you would take the best care of that vehicle you possibly could. You would buy the best gas, get the highest grade oil changes and frequent oil changes. You would ensure proper maintenance, doing everything you could possibly do to take care of that one car, because that's it - you have it for life. Why is it any different with our bodies?

That has stuck with me. Now I treat food as fuel. A treat for me no longer has to be food. A treat for me is going out and buying new clothes. A treat for me means I don't have to drive to a big and tall specialty store that doesn't even have a size big enough for me. A treat for me is being able to wear normal clothes. A treat for me is not having to have my seat all the way back and the sunroof cover open to fit my head. A treat for me is being able to go on trips, in an airplane or rent a car. A treat for me is getting up out of bed that isn't a mattress on the floor. A treat for me is sitting on a couch that isn't bent in the middle and looking like a banana. A treat for me is sitting in a booth at a restaurant. A treat for me is fitting in a movie seat, a dentists chair or even a hospital bed. A treat for me is getting up in the morning now and being able to go for a walk without feeling out of breath and enjoying the scenery that's around me.

Food doesn't have to be a reward. Why does food always have to be a reward? Why can't other things be a reward? Food should just be fuel.

To me that means eating fruit; eating a lot more vegetables; eating lean, not fatty meats. Food as fuel means getting up in the morning and having a nice big, healthy breakfast to get my body and my metabolism engaged. That gives my body energy. That keeps my body in the best condition it can be. What I put in is what I get out. I honestly believe that old cliché, "garbage in, garbage out." I also believe in, "healthy in, healthy out!"

I'm glad I can have delicious, healthy food. I eat great. I eat delicious things all the time. In the morning, I'll have a nice healthy omelet. There's nothing wrong with it or unhealthy about it and it's really tasty. I eat fish, chicken and veggies. I eat fruit. If I find a nice, delicious apple, I look at that the same way now as I used to look at a piece of cake. That's all I need to get a taste of sweetness. It's all just a matter of adjusting your mentality.

The Mind — Central to a change of lifestyle, *the mind* is a very powerful thing. The same mind that can take me or you and tell us that we can train and we can climb a mountain, or the mind that will tell us we can walk for miles and miles is the same mind that will convince you that you're useless and that you don't belong anywhere except on the end of the couch eating yourself into oblivion or into a coma.

Our minds need to be retrained. We have to stop looking at food with a reward or comfort mentality.

Let me say it again. Change your mind. Stop thinking we deserve or need junk food. If you get rid of the junk, the processed sugar and the pop, and start walking I'm convinced you've got nine tenths of your battle won right there.

Energy — I find that since I changed my diet, I sleep less, but I constantly wake up full of energy. Before, I slept a lot longer and I woke up feeling unrested and very sluggish. Whereas now I have energy right away, as soon as I wake up. Now I can go to bed for four or five hours of sleep, wake up and feel I'm good to go. I think a lot of that has to do with food as fuel, the food itself energizes me. The empty sugar calories of junk food in the evening used to suck the life out me overnight and I used to be tired all the time. Now my body is getting the nutrition it needs every single day. I know I'm supposed to get more sleep than that, but when I do wake up, it doesn't matter. Even with 4 or 5 hours of sleep I'm totally energized and ready to go.

I really don't know the science behind a lot of it. I'm not an expert. I understand that some complex carbohydrates are good in some ways when they are nutritious. I also know that sugar or too much bread and pasta, "empty" calories as they call them, are useless fillers. They might feel good for a minute while I taste them in my mouth and maybe I feel good for a few minutes afterwards with the sugar high, but then a bit later I feel drained and miserable. The sugar rush has no nutritional value to actually *fuel* my body. It gets me down mentally too as I think, "I shouldn't have eaten that." I would feel tired and sluggish and the medical issues would start and the worry would grow especially when I was not living a highly active lifestyle. I obviously knew that I should have been staying away from all those carbs.

Natural — I believe that we need to eat in a more *natural* way. This is one concept that I hope we can all agree on. Call it Mother Nature or God's way — it doesn't matter what your believe or how we got here. Regardless of our belief systems, the world didn't come to a point where it "naturally" began to produce cheesecake, chocolate bars, chips and candy. Those are manmade inventions. The world came with fruit. It came with vegetables. It came with beans and nuts and seeds. It came with all of these *natural, unprocessed* foods. That's all I really knew to start this journey — I had to eat naturally.

I've come to the realization that I had to stay away from the *fake* food. I'll never touch it again. It's been two and a half years and I haven't had a bite of sugar of any kind. I've had very little bread and limited potatoes. I'm also very careful with rice and starches. For me, I had to totally get away from the junk food and desserts. The longer I've been away from processed sugar, the less I crave it. Both pop and diet pop are horrible for your health.

I don't know if there is any scientific support for this, but I found that when I drank a lot of diet pop, it just gave me cravings. I couldn't satisfy those cravings. I would get up in the morning and have a diet cola at 5:00 o'clock in the morning. As soon as I started drinking diet pop, I was craving all kinds of junk food. The more junk food I ate, the more diet pop I wanted. I remember reading an article about how diet soda kind of tricks the stomach into believing that it's having something sweet. I was drinking a ton of that stuff.

I remember when I first came back from the evacuation, I had a case of twenty four diet soda in my fridge. That pop was still waiting for me, nice and cold. Any other time in my life that would have been like finding gold in my fridge, because I had forgotten all about it. I threw the whole case right out, I remember it clearly. Those diet sugars, they taste like candy, but it's killing us from the inside out. The caffeine isn't helping either.

The New Breakfast — My breakfasts now are fairly healthy. I eat bacon once every couple weeks; not a big portion, maybe once or twice a month. I cook eggs with a little bit of cheese and pepper. I used to get into trouble in the old days with the hash browns fried up in all that butter and all that toast. I don't do that any more, just eggs.

If I'm on a day off, I'll get up in the morning, I'll make an omelet with a bit of cheese and some mushrooms and enjoy a banana or an apple. I always have apples and bananas on hand. I'll fry up two or three eggs if I don't make an omelet.

Donut/Coffee Shops — I still love to head to the coffee shop. I drink coffee, either black or half a cream. I don't touch any donuts. I still go to Tim Hortons. I love their coffee; no donuts, Timbits, muffins or bagels of any kind. I do, however, get their chilli. I love Tim Hortons chilli. I always say no to the bread. They'll say to me, "Well, it's included in the meal," but I don't eat it!

For me, the bread would just go in the garbage and I don't like wasting food. I'm not going to eat it, so, I just say "No bread, thanks!"

Restaurants and Home Cooking — If I can go into a donut shop and find something relatively healthy, I have learned I can go to *any* restaurant and I can always find something to eat that's pretty healthy, not perfect, but good enough to lose 337 pounds in this new lifestyle in less than two years. People will always make excuses, and say that no one can eat healthy at a restaurant. Sure we can!

The first thing we see on a restaurant menu are usually the appetizers, nachos, deep-fried mozzarella sticks, all kinds of greasy stuff pulling at our attention. If we keep reading, we'll see soups, salads and some types of entrées that are just meat and vegetables. That's where we simply have to make a better choice. We don't have to get the French Fries just because "it comes with it." We can ask for veggies instead or a side salad. It might cost an extra dollar or two, but we're worth it! Sometimes I will just pick a healthy salad. I never get desert. If I really feel I need something sweet, I'll grab an apple at home.

I enjoy cooking at home now. I try not to eat out too much. As I mentioned earlier if I'm on a day off, for breakfast I'll make an omelet with fruit or eggs and fruit. I don't use salt and I'll fry it up in a pan lightly sprayed. I don't use butter or oil. I use the olive oil cooking spray, or I like the coconut oil spray. I'm always an early riser. I'm up early, then I'll go for a walk.

At lunchtime I love to go to Tim Hortons for the chilli I just mentioned. I love my coffee and chilli lunch. During the day I might go for another walk. I might go for a little drive. The difference is now I don't drive to fast food places. I'll drive and maybe go try on some clothes. I'll run some errands. I'll go for a walk through the mall. I'll go to the park and just go for a walk, maybe see somebody I know, hang out and chat for a while.

In the summertime there's a park in Fort McMurray that I love going to. It's right on the Snye river. It's a beautiful area, where lots of families gather. There are hundreds of people down by the water. There's a beach volleyball court. There's a nice hill where you can sit on the grass, you can walk the beautiful trails. I enjoy that very much, walking and enjoying the beauty. Before I would drive around and go to different fast food restaurants. Now I enjoy this beautiful piece of nature.

For supper on my days off I usually buy something fresh every day. I love to explore the fresh groceries, find unfrozen, unseasoned chicken, or maybe a piece of salmon, or a steak — some spectacular Alberta beef. I enjoy adding a nice salad, or I might boil up some veggies; a turnip, a couple of carrots, whatever vegetable I feel like. I also like to put a roast in the slow cooker all day.

There are a couple of places in Fort McMurray where I like to eat that are really healthy in the event that I don't feel like cooking. There's lots of restaurants I can go to and order healthy options, but there are two spots that are just plain healthy and clean. There's a place called "Eat Clean." They have a great menu and also do pre-made meals to go, like chicken, fish, steak, usually with broccoli or other veggies; excellent healthy options. I don't go there often because I prefer to cook for myself at home, but those are great healthy meals to take to work, much better than the old fast foods I used to pig out with.

Another spot I love is Freshii, it's a chain with hundreds of locations in cities in many countries. They have fresh ingredients for salads, soups, wraps and bowls - many wonderful healthy, fresh options. I never would have guessed it a few years ago, but these are the kind of "fast food" places I head to nowadays.

I'll have my evening meal around 5:00 o'clock or 5:30, and that's all I will eat until the next morning. If I'm still hungry at night, if I feel I *really* need something I'll have an apple. I'll eat that and remember years before how I'd inhale a big bag of chips, some ice-cream and chocolate. It's a different day!

If I find a nice juicy apple, that does the trick. Sometimes the boys will bring me fruit at work where they used to bring me chips and junk food. It's funny! What a change! It's a whole new lifestyle.

That's my day. It doesn't revolve around food anymore, it revolves around living and food merely fuels my new lifestyle. I'm always full of energy. Apparently instead of spending the night hours struggling to digest sugar and carbs and whatever greasy thing I had for supper, my body has already processed that hours before I sleep. Now my body can rest and repair itself overnight. Eating before bed is hard on the body — I am glad I can give it a real rest now.

If I'm *really* hungry at night, I also drink water. It takes away the cravings, it takes away the hunger and fills me right up.

Last week, on the road, we went to a restaurant while we were in the U.S.A., an Applebee's. It was my first time ever in that restaurant. Pretty much any restaurant you go to they'll always have a few healthy choices. I had a bowl of French onion soup, and a Thai salad. Anything you have, there'll always be some stuff in there that's probably not the healthiest, but I picked the healthiest choice I could find. That entire meal came to about 800 calories. I eat healthy at home, but I always do fine in restaurants now too.

Travel Snacks — Even when I'm traveling. I can usually find something at many gas stations. These days a lot of gas stations sell fruit. Many times I've been able to get a banana, an apple, a black coffee, a bottle of water, nuts; there are good options. You don't have to get chocolate bars, ice cream or packaged baked goods just because they are there on display. We can still make healthy choices. I eat a lot of nuts. I try to find packages that are high in protein and low in sodium.

I find I can also be really smart if I'm going to be travelling, I can think ahead a bit and buy snacks before I travel, a few apples, bananas, my go-to snacks, some water and a coffee.

Then I'm not "forced" to eat fast food, not that I ever am, but I want to do what I can to avoid getting dragged down.

Even while we were working on this book over in the States, I saw a Dunkin' Donuts and remembered that I had always wanted to try their coffee. We popped in and I ordered my extra large with half a cream and sitting right there on the counter were a couple bananas for sale! I grabbed both of those. I had one right then with my coffee and had one later back at the hotel. Who would have know that fruit was available in a donut shop? The coffee was delicious by the way!

There's really no need for excuses anymore. It's all about making healthy choices and many stores and restaurants offer healthy options if I'm not too lazy to notice.

Late Night Snacks — These days I almost feel guilty if I have a single apple at 9:00 p.m.; like I've indulged or binged. Now that I know new limits, an apple at night is pushing it a bit. Never again will I be excessive. No more "treats" for this dawg! Instead, it's nice to go for a walk at 9:00 or 10:00 p.m. rather than binging. It's a much healthier choice!

Grocery Stores — I stay away from junk food, especially sugar. I stay away from many of those beef snacks and jerky, because they're filled with sodium and it's usually highly processed food. I try to eat as much fresh food as I can. That's why when I'm home, I'll go to the grocery store, usually every third day, to try to get fresh fruits, veggies and meat.

A tip I've heard since I've been eating clean food is that the best way to shop for groceries is to search the outer aisles. I heard it was wise to stay away from the interior aisles. I thought about it and it makes sense. The outer aisles are where you find the fruit, the vegetables, then maybe the bakery, which I skip obviously, but then the meat, the dairy, eggs and the fish counter. I shop for all the fresh *outside aisle* foods. If it's not fresh, it's meant to have a longer shelf life (the inside aisles) which makes salt and other preservatives necessary.

The new lifestyle means shopping the outside aisles. Years ago I was making poor choices on the inside aisles, pop and chips, snacks, cakes and sugar. I suppose these changes truly have happened from the *inside out*.

Sodium — Good old fashioned "salt" and all it's other names (sodium, MSG, baking soda) should not be entering our bodies more than 2000 mg per day. Less is better.

Fruit and Veggies — Did I mention I eat apples and bananas? I do. I eat a ton of apples and bananas. If I can go find a nice, big, ripe, juicy apple now, I feel like I've got it made.

Fuji apples are my favourite. I really like any variety of apples, except for rotten apples. I'll eat any kind of apple and enjoy it. In Fort McMurray, all our apples come in from British Columbia and they're gorgeous. Granted, they are expensive. It's common to pay $12 or $13 for a bag of apples. I will go to the big box stores to get them cheaper, but they are still $9 a bag. Fort McMurray has been ranked the most expensive city in Canada to live, especially in boom times. Housing prices have come down since 2015, but groceries are still expensive. Junk food is expensive too though, so I might as well eat a delicious, sweet, juicy apple if I do want something sweet. It also keeps doctors away.

I know there are a lot of diets out there that say you have to stay away from fruit, especially if you're diabetic. However, the thing that has really helped me is just eating naturally. I understand that if you are diabetic or even eating keto, they say you can have any type of berry; strawberries, blue berries, black berries, raspberries; anything that has the word *berry* in the name is fine and not too high in sugar. I mostly eat bananas and apples and I don't overdo it.

I enjoy those raw veggie trays from the grocery store, those are great. That's how I eat a lot of my vegetables.

My love for apples and bananas, has spread beyond my

own home. It's funny because people that I will go to visit now or when I go home and see mom, the one thing they all know is that they have to have bananas on hand. I'm a low-maintenance guest if there are bananas on hand.

No More Junk Food — It's literally been two and a half years since I had a bag of chips, a chocolate bar, ice cream or a piece of cake. I'm truly done with junk food and I will never go back to it again. For me there's no way I'll have a "cheat day" once a week, or even once a month. I can't. I'm just eating clean, natural and cutting out the junk once and for all! I'm not just cutting *down*, but I've entirely cut it *OUT!*

I didn't change my lifestyle with a special fad diet or something that cost me money. There were no pills, or surgery; no kind of fat farm or spa treatments; no drops; no supplements of any kind. I've just been losing weight based on an internal shift when something clicked during the evacuation. I stopped lying to myself, I stopped putting it off and I just did it. Then once I got through the first three weeks of lifestyle change and the scale indicated that I had lost thirty pounds, the momentum shifted and I decided to never go back to that old lie, that old story, that old me, that old Tony who was lonely and miserable. Never. Ever. Again.

Now that I've eliminated the junk and lost all the weight, for the first time I will have limited amounts of carbs. I have to know my limit and stay within it. I could have a little pasta now, I have a little bread now, a few times a year. Every once in a while if I have a salad and it comes with garlic bread, if I know it's very delicious I will have a piece.

My birthday is in January. I'll usually go to my favourite steakhouse, the Keg and the bread they bring out before the meal is my cake. I don't need cake. I don't need junk food, but I will have a few pieces of bread each year now.

I'll eat probably a couple of those things, once a year, but, generally, no bread, no pasta, not on a regular basis. I'll have rice if it's the only option. Just a few days ago, I'd had a full day and I didn't feel like cooking the night before I flew out, so I went to Moxie's Grill where I had some grilled chicken. The plate came out with a huge tree of broccoli on it. The other side was wild rice and I enjoyed that; a delicious, healthy supper.

I've been getting away from decades of life-ruining habits the longer I've been away from junk food and processed sugar. I picture a person in a boat and the further they row away from land, the less they see of it. The less they see of that land, they find less desire to turn back towards it and eventually they are just as glad to be on another shore. With this new lifestyle, with how I eat now, I want to keep going towards that goal. The further I get away from sugar and junk food, the less and less I want it.

It doesn't even bother me now to be with people who are eating junk food. I don't crave a thing. This new shore I'm living on, I don't even see that old land, that old way of eating, that old way of living. I can't even imagine getting back into that old way of life eating sugar and junk; it feels disgusting to me. Even to think about having one bite of something is repulsive.

I've found two things about this: (i) Physically I don't crave it, whether that's because I gave up pop, diet pop or I gave up sugar, I don't crave it any more. I just don't desire it, but also, (ii) I remember the pain of that life like it was yesterday. That pain has caused me to look at that junk food not as a pleasure, but I look at it with *hatred* because of how it ruined my life. It took away the life that I'm enjoying now. I look at cake and if I could punch it in the mouth, I would. It's sickening to me.

Body Needs — Healthy eating, like that meal I just mentioned from Moxie's, it's not heavy. It's just what the body *needs*. You don't feel like you need to go and have a two-hour nap afterwards, weighted down with empty calories. When healthy food is fuel, when you're done eating, you feel energized. For example, at Swiss Chalet I get the double leg chicken dinner that started me off on this journey; chicken with the skin removed and veggies. It's like gasoline to my body's energy system. It doesn't seem wise to follow my shallow desires for sugar. My body needs more than that.

Either you're going to give into your cravings, or you're going to give into what your body needs; fuel or pleasure! The way I look at it is if you give your body the essentials that it needs, it will give you the life that you want. I shared an analogy earlier. Treat your body like a car, give it the best fuel and your body will run like a finely tuned machine!

Once in a while, I will have potatoes, but I won't overdo it. The traditional combination of meat and potatoes, especially a large portion of spuds is a recipe for needing a nap, so I don't often have potatoes. Maybe once a month, or every six weeks I will have a portion of potatoes. If I view food as fuel, too many potatoes is more like putting water in my gas tank.

I will eat sweet potatoes. I'll eat all the veggies, turnips, carrots; I love those great big carrots, they're huge, the size of my forearm almost. Last week. I cooked a roast, with big carrots, and turnips. As I alway do, instead of using salt to season the roast, I added an onion to give it some flavour. I let it cook for seven or eight hours until it was very tender. Sometimes for dessert I'll have an apple or some other piece of fruit after a meal like that. If I go for an evening walk, usually when I come back, I'll eat a banana. A couple of bananas for the day is usually my limit.

With my limited knowledge of diet and exercise, all I knew for sure was that junk food was terrible. I was tired of having so much of it. Let's be honest, I knew all along that it was horrible for my health and my weight. You would have to be lying to yourself not to acknowledge that.

"No more junk food and start walking." There's my big fancy secret. It's not rocket science!

As I said earlier, I had tried to diet *hundreds* of times over the years. I wouldn't make it through the day and I'd say, "I've done well. I deserve a bit of ice cream."

One carton of ice cream later I would say, "Actually, I will start tomorrow." It seems kind of funny to say it now, but that's exactly what I would do. I was only kidding myself. To be honest, there were days that I wouldn't make it through an hour and then I'd talk myself into a "treat" and just keep the addiction cycle rolling.

I saw on social media people would go have a treat day, or a cheat day once every four or five days, once a week, once every two weeks, or once a month. Other people would go on certain programs where points would allow them to have a treat, but in the end it was this puppy mentality that said, "I deserve a treat." Like puppies, all we are training ourselves for is an addiction to sugar, salt and carbs.

I've realized I just can't do that any longer. For me, I had to go a different route. If I wanted to get this off this nightmare of an obesity roller-coaster ride, I decided, once and for all, I could never touch that junk again.

It ruined my life. I treat food like an alcoholic treats a beer. An alcoholic won't go out for a drink once a week for a "treat." He won't go to a birthday party and have half a dozen drinks because he figures, "it's only once a year." For me it was an addiction like that. I can't mess with it at all, never again. I've gone strictly cold turkey on junk food; complete junk food abstinence. There are some things in life, there are some points that you get to in where you just have to say like I did, "I can't have that again. Ever. I need to draw the line there. I want to have a good life. I want freedom. I have to give up something to get there. I will never touch this stuff again."

I won't. I will never sample it or touch it again. My

daughter even asked me one night, she said, "Dad, when I get married, aren't you going to have any wedding cake?

I told her flat out, "No, honey, I won't." Her mother even explained it and said, "He just can't."

I'm not saying that it would cause me to gain back all the weight I lost, by having one piece of cake or one chip. I know it wouldn't. For me it's more of a mental barrier. As I consider it, it's not an issue of regaining weight, it's all the bad memories that are associated with it.

I want nothing to do with it.

I remember the pain associated with being excessively fat. I vividly remember looking at the seats I was taking up on the evacuation bus and the airplane. That's huge. It's incredibly painful. That day will always be stuck in my memories. The fire could have turned out really bad, for me, or for God knows who, because I took somebody's seat.

For me, that means no more junk food ever again; total abstinence. That was the boundary I decided on, and it worked for me. In the end, you'll never hear of anybody gaining weight eating apples. You might have heard they kept the doctor away with apples, but not gained weight! When was the last time you ever heard of anybody getting obese from having two apples a day? If that's your treat, an apple, a cup of berries, or a banana, as long as you are eating healthy, why not have one or two portions of those a day?

As I began eating cleaner and healthier, my no-junk-food-and-walking plan, I picked up some other concepts along the way. People at work or other people that I came across who were into nutrition and exercise would pass along tips that had worked for them. That's where I heard the idea about shopping clean visiting the outside aisles at a grocery store selecting real and living foods. I learned more about eating healthier by staying away from the middle aisles. That's also where I learned to stay away from processed foods and especially salty prepared foods. They might save you time in the short term, but in the long term, those salty meals, especially frozen dinners are hurting you.

Cook it Yourself — I've also learned to cook as much food for myself as possible, rather than prepared foods, fast foods or take-out. Foods might look fresh in that beautiful packaging, but they're often stored with high amounts of sodium or sugar. That was a really good tip that helped me.

Selecting and preparing your own unseasoned, unpreserved meats and vegetables lets you be the boss in the amount of sodium and sugar involved. If you're the cook you can choose zero sodium and sugar if you wish!

Water — I've dropped over three hundred pounds, but I haven't been drinking like a fish. I know that a lot of people say that the biggest key to losing weight is drinking plenty of water and yes, it's very good for you, but I've been getting most of my hydration from eating lots of fruits and vegetables. I get water from my coffee too, as I've said I drink it black, that is sort of like water. I know it's bad. I'm trying to drink more water. I know I should.

My point is, I'm not doing everything right. I'm definitely not doing everything perfectly. However, I do think, for me and probably for most people in the world, cutting all the junk food out of your diet and consistently going for walks will absolutely change your life!!

I don't want to say that anyone needs to defy medical studies. I'm simply trying to illustrate that I don't know everything. I know very little and that limited knowledge has been enough common sense to change my life. There's been lots of research and information that's been written and it's wonderful. My only point is, if you're waiting to learn to know everything before you get started, maybe you should reconsider and just start with the obvious?

Earlier in the book I mentioned my friend Lisa Bapty

whose mom gave me $300 to move out west. Lisa's husband Thomas, he's an American, a military guy, who's really into exercise and healthy eating. I've learned a lot from him. He said, "It is amazing that you've lost all that weight drinking as little water as you do."

When it comes down to it, I just did the obvious. We all know what to do. Maybe we just need to do it!

Walking — Truthfully, I now walk a lot in the course of a day, I usually walk about an average of an hour a day, just by moving around at work from one place to another. I'm burning about five or six hundred calories right there. I'm fortunate that I don't have to sit at a desk all day.

Something I appreciate about walking is that there are sidewalks everywhere. I can walk anywhere. There are trails, paths, parks and road sides everywhere in the world. Walking is very easy and doable. I love my walks. I enjoy the time. It clears my head. I'll talk to myself, think about things and even pray a little bit as I walk. I enjoy the fresh air. I like to discover different trails.

Fort McMurray has a lot of beautiful trails, trails that I never knew they had until I set out to walk. Now I'm discovering a whole new world. There's one trail in Fort McMurray right downtown that's neat. It goes right along the river and there's a lot of native art on the trail. There are foxes, wolves and various sculptured animals painted by different schools. There are different native sculptures hidden in the trees. It's really cool. I've been in Fort McMurray 19 years and just discovered a lot of this culture in the last three years since I started walking.

I mentioned how recently in Calgary I parked the car at the hotel, took a cab downtown and toured all around downtown on foot. Walking is a perfect way to explore a city. I couldn't do that years ago. In Calgary I was able to check out buildings and museums that I had never seen before.

On average right now, outside of work I walk anywhere between three to five kilometres each day. I usually set goals that are distance-based. I started off my walks originally as time-based walks; five minutes, then six, then seven, but then as I lost weight I got faster. I get up in the morning and if I'm working a day shift I'll get up at 4:30 a.m. and do a 3.5 to 4.5 kilometre walk. Returning to the condo I'll make my breakfast and then get ready for work. When I'm working the night shift I'll do the same distance before work. On my days off I have more time. I'll often walk six or eight kilometres those days. I might take two walks a day. I'll do that every day for a while and then take two walks a day every third day. Then I might take a break and just walk once a day. I'll take a day where I won't walk at all just to rest up a little bit. I like to mix it up. I like to hop in the car to explore a different trail in other parts of town. I like variety. I love walking when I'm on vacation too, seeing new places. Thing always look different from the walking perspective and I see places I never would have seen when I explore on foot.

A New Chapter with Emma — If I'm out with Emma, we'll still go to a movie and she'll have her popcorn. Popcorn is not too bad for you, but I still don't touch it. Not only will I not touch junk food as such, I won't touch anything that even looks like junk food. I just stay away from the whole thing. I could have popcorn with no butter on it. It's actually not too bad, but for me I feel, "What's the point? Why eat popcorn without butter? That's just wrong." When I used to get popcorn, I would get butter halfway through, then the rest of the butter on top. I would buy a pack of M&Ms (known as "flavour boosters" in select theatres in Canada), pour the candy on the popcorn (the warm popcorn melts the chocolate a bit), shake it all around, then add more butter. That was my movie habit. Now, I don't need any of it.

I'm trying to be a good example for Emma these days

knowing I definitely haven't been over the years. I don't force the things I eat on her. We definitely don't have dessert as much as we used to. In the old days, three years ago, I'd always make sure she had dessert and treats during a date. Now when we go to restaurants I never get dessert anymore, so many times she doesn't have it either.

Emma loves Montana's BBQ and Bar. When I go to Montana's, I have the skillet full of veggies and meat for the fajitas. Most times I'll just have the meat and veggies, but I might have a tortilla wrap sometimes, but not often. I'll also get the grilled chicken with the veggies, at her favourite spot. There are always healthy options even at a BBQ restaurant.

Early to Rise — There is one other good tip that I find has helped me. I like to get up early in the morning. In terms of fuel, the most important meal of the day for me is breakfast. I like to start my body off on the right foot. I love to get up early in the morning and have a healthy protein breakfast which is most often eggs. Then I still have a full day in front of me to eat healthy food. I have my breakfast, my lunch, my supper.

There's a psychological edge in getting up early. If I get up early in the morning, I'm more likely to go to bed early at night near 9:00 o'clock. The cravings at night, that desire for a midnight snack doesn't show up if I've already been sleeping for a few hours. I used to get "food boredom" I would call it at night. I used to eat because I was bored, or watch a movie and want a late night snack. If I go to bed earlier at night, I have less opportunity to get in trouble in the evening.

I usually try to eat my evening meal around 5 PM. I usually go to bed around 9:00/9:30, because that's when I'm getting tired. When I get up early, I only have that window from six to nine o'clock in the evening where I've got to be really disciplined; instead of having that window from 6:00 PM until 2:00 in the morning. That's deadly.

I'm always hungry at night. I think the old habits of wanting to eat junk food at night is a hard one to kick. Sitting down to watch a movie years ago, it was easy for me to get pulled into a bag of chips and dip, some ice cream and a chocolate bar. That was my old life, those were my old habits. These days I don't watch a lot of TV. I'm more likely to go for a walk so the TV and munchie cravings aren't an issue.

It a simple concept that works for me that if I get up early in the morning, I'm more likely to go to bed early at night and avoid snack craving time. Night time for a lot of people is the hardest time that they fight against the temptation of eating junk food. Early to rise and early to bed helped me a lot.

I have come to understand that it's just not smart for me to eat anything at night. Sleeping keeps me out of trouble.

A Guaranteed Fail — I find my life changed dramatically when I started to stay away from processed sugar or the artificial sweeteners. I find aspartame only gave me cravings for junk food. I avoid all of that, all together. It seems when people put weight back on, something they all have in common is that they went back to eating junk food, it's a guaranteed diet fail. I still get sugar through the fruit I eat. Processed sugar, that white stuff that comes in five pound bags of death, it's very unhealthy. I might not be able to avoid it in everything, but I don't put it on anything. I avoid processed sugar and I avoid junk food. I stay away from it. The longer I've stayed away, the less I crave it.

I'm done with it all. No junk food, no chips, no chocolate bars, no cheese cake, no fast food, no French Fries. It's pretty obvious. I'm not trying to write a diet book. It's really just common sense.

I know I've had to take a strong stand, a line in the sand with no sugar and no junk at all. It wouldn't be enough for me to say, "Okay, just on my birthday I'm going to have a piece of ice-cream cake." For me I had to go cold turkey. That's because

I had to treat it like an alcoholic. It was killing me. An alcoholic does not celebrate his birthday by saying, "I'm going have shots tonight! Whoo-hoo. It's cheat night!"

When an alcoholic gives up drinking, they give it up entirely. They determine that they can never touch alcohol again. I'm always going to be a food-oholic. I can't cheat once a week, once every two weeks. I was addicted to food, to be honest. I looked to food too often for comfort when I was lonely, or for fun and feeling good when I was bored. I was totally addicted. Now, I just can't touch it.

I'm not saying everybody has to be as drastic as I was. Obviously, if a guy only has to lose 20 or 30 pounds, sure, he could probably have a piece of cake once in a while. For me though, where it almost took my life, I had to take it very seriously.

No matter where you are in terms of needing to lose weight, let me encourage you with this thought once again. You don't have to be a prisoner to food. You don't have to be a prisoner to the situation you're in. This is going to sound awfully cliché, but you only really fail if you truly give up. Keep trying! Whether it takes you ten, a hundred or a thousand attempts, it doesn't matter. Just please don't give up. You don't need junk food like you think you do. You can survive without it. You will actually *prosper* without it.

Seasons — I love the heat now. I froze to death all the time three years ago. I love the heat down in Mexico, but I also love winter now too. Let me contrast the seasons for you, not summer and winter but the old and the new seasons of three years ago and today.

Wintertime was probably the hardest season for me. The wintertime was really stressful and that's when I would probably end up eating even more. I drove to work all the time. Every day in the wintertime I was watching the weather because I was worried about poor driving conditions. To this day I hate driving on winter roads if it's snowing or if it's slippery. When I was huge I had no choice. I had to drive to work. I was too big to take the bus work provided.

I had that Chrysler 300 and it was a rear-wheel drive car. If the night before work I knew it was going to be snowing the next morning, I was very stressed because I knew I'd have to drive 26 km in that rear-wheel drive, the whole back end was going to be fishtailing. People would be passing me on the highway in their big Alberta pick-up trucks and all-wheel drive vehicles while I'm just spinning out, fishtailing my way along to work.

It was very stressful and I kept thinking if I fishtailed off the highway and got in an accident, how would they get me out of the car? If I do get to the hospital somehow, how are they going to deal with me? If I have to be off work for a while, how am I going to deal with that? All of that worry would constantly go through my head. I would get to work, where onsite in the wintertime it would often drop to minus 30 or minus 35. I'd be wearing those flimsy old shoes with the Velcro. I'd have no socks on, a thin pair of gym pants that are very light, nothing underneath, just boxers, an old summer t-shirt, basically a golf shirt because that's all I can get to fit me and a size 6X coat that's not even a winter coat, it's just a fall jacket really that I can't get closed or zip up.

I'd finally get to work, already stressed out. At work I'd park my vehicle but I'd have to get out there pretty early because I couldn't walk very far so I'd have to get there early enough to find a really good parking spot close to the entrance. I'd have to get out in the cold and pretend it didn't bother me. I'd head through security to the gate. They have these big turnstiles, almost like a cattle gates designed for normal sized people. I'd swipe my card and spin my way through. I'd wriggle through those barriers trying not to get stuck.

As I'd be walking through hundreds of people would be

coming into work the same time as me. Suncor's a huge company, with hundreds of people starting each shift at the same time. Many of them would be staring at me. I hated being in public. Once I was through the gate all of us would have to wait for the shuttle bus to take us down to the mine. I'd have to get on that bus. There'd be dozens of other people waiting to get on the bus. I'd be in this line up, but I'd have to wait for a special seat with enough room, so what I would do if the bus was packed or close to being packed, I'd let the bus leave and I would stand outside in the cold for a bit longer and wait for the next bus. I didn't want to get on a full bus and have to share a seat with somebody. The next bus would soon pull up and I would get on and go right to the very back seat. Anybody coming on, wouldn't have to sit with me or walk past me judging me because I was taking up too much room up front. I would go back there and just sit back and avoid all of that. If it meant freezing outside a little longer to avoid the judgemental looks, so be it.

All the bus drivers kind of knew me, so normally they would wait for the bus to fill up, but if they looked in the rearview mirror to check the bus and the only empty seat was next to me, they would close the door and pull away knowing I couldn't share that empty seat beside me. The bus would then head off to the transfer point about a five minute drive past security where I had to switch to another bus that would take us all down to the mine. Suncor is huge so they've got buses going to the mine, to the plant and to different spots on this massive property.

I'd have to do all this over again on the second bus to reach the mine. I'd get to the transfer point, walk up to another bus stop and wait. If the bus was half full, even at minus 30 outside, I still wouldn't get on that bus. Even though it's only half full, there's a chance that there's already one person in each seat and there's no open seat by itself. I needed an open seat for myself, so I would wait outside, minus 30, minus 35 in my thin velcro shoes and open jacket, nearly frozen to death. The next bus would come along. I would get on that bus and go to the very back of the bus again avoiding people and their gaze. Then at the end of the day, I'd do that all that over in the other direction, going back up to the gate.

All day long if it was snowing I'd constantly be looking at the weather reports and if it was continually snowing throughout the day, I would have a lot of anxiety because of what I was going to face after work. I'd get to my car and sit in the car knowing I have to drive home in this weather. I would let my car warm up for a while and then I would continue waiting for most of the traffic to go so I could get on the highway without having a line up of vehicles behind me.

Having lots of room on the highway, with no one tailgating me was important to me; driving slowly would give me room to relax, let me drive at my own pace, do my own thing. I'd let everybody else go first and I would go last. I would take my time driving home. In those winter months, especially if the weather was bad, after finishing work at 8:00, I'd get home sometimes at 9:15, even 9:30.

When I got home I'd be stressed out from the winter driving. I would not have eaten much all day because I couldn't. As you know, bathroom size was an issue for me at work. I just didn't want to use the bathrooms at all at work because of how big I was. It was all very embarrassing for me.

Arriving home, I wouldn't have really eaten much all day. I'd eaten a lot of calories in the morning but not much by way of food volume. Throughout the day I might have brought in a lunch bag: three or four Diet Pepsi's and a bag of chips or a chocolate bar or some little treat I'd have gotten at Tim Hortons in the morning. I'd eat that during the day but feel like I was starving at the end of the day.

On the way home, I'd get into Fort McMurray and near

where I live there are all kinds of fast food spots I could visit. I'd drive up to KFC and I'd order at the drive-thru. I didn't want to get out of the car. I'd get a 10-piece bucket. I'd head home and I'd seven pieces on my couch. Before I'd go to bed, I'd slam down some junk food out of my fridge and cupboards saving three pieces of chicken for the next day, but I wouldn't eat those. I'd just give it away at work. I was the 600-pound KFC fairy giving out thighs, wings and drumsticks.

That was my routine throughout the winter. I hated the winter.

Things are different these days. I have a totally different attitude about winter. I put a post up on Facebook the other day that reminded me of how different winter is. It was a picture of me in a winter coat.

When I was back home last summer, my dad gave me this brand new winter jacket, size large, one of those goose down-filled jackets. I'd wanted one of those jackets, a little dream of mine. I used to see people wearing those for years, a full winter jacket, a proper warm coat that would close and fasten properly. They didn't make the goose down-filled jacket sized 7X; too many geese would go bald for that. My dad never wore it. My mom gave it to him for Christmas a couple years ago, but it just wasn't his thing. He gave it to me when I was home. These days when it snows in Fort McMurray 10 or 20 centimetres and it's cold, that doesn't bother me at all. I think back to a few years ago of how cold I was, how many shuttle buses I had to wait for, nearly frozen to death and I smile when I think of it. I smile, grinning from ear to ear I'm sure. I don't have to face that anymore. My car's nice and warm parked down in the underground parking. It doesn't have to be used. It's protected, nestled away in the carpark. I don't have to worry about driving to work.

I get up in the morning, go for a walk first then make a nice breakfast. I see the weather report, I see the snow outside and I am stress free; even if I see the forecast for the week and it's says it'll be snowing for four or five consecutive days and I know the roads are going to be horrible. I just smile. I say, "Bring it on, Old Man Winter!"

I get up in the morning and I get ready to step outside on my *bridge*, I easily pull my nice big brown winter boots on over my socks and I smile. I tie them up tight and I smile again as I think back to those old Velcro shoes with no socks. Then I put on that big warm goose-down-filled winter jacket, (only size large), I do the zipper up, with all kinds of room to spare. I have a nice shirt on underneath. I put my hat on, my toque, my mitts. Life is good. I'm smiling.

I could get mitts and hats before, sizes that would fit, but the way I thought before was mitts and a toque aren't going to help too much if my coat's wide open. So if I was going to be frozen, I was really going to be frozen. Now I smile. You can't beat that. When it snows, I can't wipe the smile off my face because right away I'm reminded that even though it's wintertime, I don't have any anxiety to face and I don't have to be cold any more. For years I lived that miserable winter routine. I used to despise October and November. I used to dread those months and what was coming. Now I'm smiling all the way as I walk to the bus stop. I couldn't take the bus before, but now I walk to the bus stop grinning.

The Suncor bus stop is not far from my house. The buses work provides for the employees are wonderful, big, warm beautiful buses, air conditioned in the summer, cozy and warm in the winter. I get to the bus stop and I hear people talking and complaining as Canadians do, "I'm so cold, I hate winter, I hate the cold, I hate this snow." I'm standing there, just smiling with a stupid grin on my face.

I get on that nice warm bus. I still go to the very back seat, in the back of the bus. I sit down, I settle in and I just shake my head and I smile. I reflect on how good life is.

In the wintertime, it's always been harder for me to go see Emma because not only did I have a lot of anxiety driving just to Suncor, imagine me driving six hours to Red Deer in that cramped car with the same worries. Now I can fly there. I go online and book a short flight from Fort McMurray to Calgary, rent a car in Calgary, drive an hour up to Red Deer and it's done. No worries! I could care less about the weather. I fit in a plane and a rental car. I am no longer limited by anything.

I have another winter jacket I love. It's a nice Columbia winter jacket with a liner that goes in it. For years I used to dream of owning a Columbia jacket. I used to see people wearing them and they looked so warm. It's a size large. As soon as I could fit in that, I bought one. I paid $200 bucks for the thing. It's perfect for Alberta winters.

But now, since my father gave me the other winter coat, I just keep the lining out of the Columbia jacket and use it as a Spring travel coat because I love that jacket. It's got so many pockets and it's great for traveling. There's a selfie on Facebook if you want to see it. As I took the photo I remembered how great my life is now.

Extra Skin — They tell us that skin is actually the largest organ in the body. Now that I have lost about 340 pounds I understand that and I will tell you why. My skin has been stretched so much that now I have about **thirty** pounds of "extra" skin that I have been carrying around these recent years. It's not fat, it's just extra skin that will have to be removed surgically. When I get this extra thirty pounds of skin taken off, things are going to be even better.

I now need to get five surgeries that will cost a grand total of $65,000. This extra skin all over my body is still attached like empty burlap bags, but all of this skin used to be full of fat. I have this loose skin everywhere, not just on my stomach, but along my back, arms, legs, it's literally *everywhere* on my body where my skin has stretched. What the doctor will do is pull this skin up, pull that skin down, then my nipples will need to be readjusted to the proper place. Then they have to do another surgery to pull some other skin over. They have to do something called a "body contour" on my back, and my butt. Then they have to do my legs, and they have to renovate my arms as well.

In each surgery I have to have skin removed because it's no longer doing anything, it's extra skin that's going to die eventually. I found a doctor in Alberta who is willing to do the surgery, but it's $12,000 — $15,000 for each of the surgeries; plus tax. Who knew losing weight was going to be this expensive?

Unless you know someone who has lost a lot of weight or unless you've watched TV shows about extreme weight loss, the extra skin is something people would never really imagine. The skin had to expand when I put on those hundreds of pounds and then when I lost the weight, the skin just loses the fat but it doesn't retract as much as it's grown. It's still there. It doesn't just miraculously go away. I can never go to the gym and get that toned up or firmed up with exercise. The fat is gone but the floppy skin is all there. All of it. I'm not trying to be gross, that's just the way it is.

I recently took a vacation to visit a friend in Mexico. I still get self conscious about all of this extra skin flopping around my body. I usually just keep it tucked in and it's a reminder to me how far I've come. At the beach a lady said to me, "Take your shirt off! Go on and jump in the ocean."

"No I'm not doin' that," I said. "The Mexicans will be shooting at me. They'll be freakin' out asking 'what's that rubbery guy doing out there. Has Elastic Man or Stretch Armstrong come to our beach?' I'll just leave my shirt on for now thanks!"

A Whole New World — The contrast of the old and new season is really shocking. If I could stand up both Tony's, the old and the new, you'd be looking at Big Tony and "normal" Tony. Big Tony would be standing there and he'd be in pain simply from standing up too long. He would smile, but you would see the effects of the weight on his body. He would be completely miserable on the inside. He would have no reason to get up in the morning, nothing to look forward to, and the only happiness he would have would be his next fast food order. Then you'd have the guy that I am now. Every day there's something to look forward to! Normal Tony enjoys traveling, his income has increased, his expenses have gone down. His smile is genuine because he enjoys the happiness of being free again. He can do anything he wants.

I wish I could encourage the Tony from three years ago and tell myself that I have the strength inside of me to change. How bad do you want it? You can do it. Your life is not over Big Tony!

I can't wait to see what tomorrow holds these days. I go to bed at night excited to wake up the next day. I'm excited about work, excited about traveling, excited about seeing my daughter, excited about what the future holds, excited about meeting people and I'm excited about helping people. I'm excited about everything!

My new life these days feels like a dream. When people ask me about it, there are two images that always come to mind. One picture is being locked in a prison and finally being let out. The other image is seeing those poor souls that are handicapped in wheelchairs and imagining if they could get up and walk again and be fully healed. That's what I feel like. Those two pictures put together. I feel like a man that has been in prison for thirty years, wrongfully convicted and he's finally let out to be free. I also feel like a man that was handicapped, in a wheelchair. You know that deep down inside he just wishes he could walk again. He wishes he could be free to do whatever he has been limited with. That's what I feel like, because I handicapped myself. I put myself in that prison.

I find freedom and delight just sitting in a movie theatre seat, in a barber chair or in a restaurant booth, not spilling over the edges or getting cut in half by the table. I actually fit in there and I can put my arm on the armrest if the chair has one. Whenever I sit in a chair and I put my arm on the armrest, the fact that my stomach is not going over the side of it feels like a marvel to me.

It makes me smile. Going on a date with a woman a short while ago has been another dream come true. That would not have happened three years ago. Having people compliment me who say, "You look good," feels very warm and nice. That certainly wasn't happening three years ago. Although it might not seem like a big deal to people, the biggest thing is to me is being able to go out and just be one of the crowd. One of the things I hated the most in my former life was being singled out and being the object of constant gawking. I'm not bothered by being out in public anymore. That's something that really makes me smile. I deeply appreciate this freedom to do things that normal-sized people can do; just to be regular Tony, not to be the *big guy*. It's that little thing I love, just being a part of the crowd. It's truly wonderful.

9

No More Excuses

You can see I'm not some kind of super-dynamic guy with all kinds of clever ideas and solutions to change the weight problems of the world. I have to be the most average of average Joe's. I do hope that somehow through this simple story of mine, I can get people to realize the incredible potential they have, if they just do what they know to be true, if they set their mind to it, they can do it, whatever they need to accomplish.

There are really no good excuses not to make whatever changes you know are necessary to have a better life. I hope I've disarmed most of the lame excuses I hid behind for over a decade in the previous chapters, but let me recap a few that might still be dangling out there:

Money.

I found I didn't need money to radically change my lifestyle. Seriously.

If you can't afford some huge eating plan or detox product or pill or drops, or if you can't pay to go to the gym, don't worry. I never did. I'm sure all of those eating programs, supplements and pills and drops are helpful to some degree.

Gyms are great too, I would like to get into doing weights myself some day, but you don't need a gym membership to change your life. I never had one.

If you have a sidewalk, or even a roadside that you can walk on, that's good enough. Most sidewalks I've seen have free admission. You can lose hundreds of pounds by just walking and eating sensibly, "eating clean" as I call it, eating foods that we all know are healthy, free of sugar and salt, as fresh as possible.

I still don't know very much about diet and exercise to be honest. Common sense and things I have heard over the years taught me to lose well over 300 pounds. All I knew was to get off the sugar, get off the junk food and the fast food and get some kind of consistent exercise. It doesn't have to be running or training for marathons or some heroic sports thing. I just had to walk for goodness sake!

Eureka!

"Well, Tony, it's easy for you to say all this, you had this big life awakening moment on the airplane and on the bus. I've never had that."

Everybody has their bus moments, their airplane moments; moments of complete and utter shame, frustration or embarrassment. It doesn't have to be a bus. It could be anything that helps you lock in on your goal and go for it. Let me be honest. From previous chapters you know about other times where I **should have** had life awakening moments, but I never did. I blew it. I knew how wonderful life could have been, but I wasted all those years. I should've lost this weight a long time ago.

Procrastination.

Let me say this once again: you only get one life. There are those of us who believe in the afterlife, obviously, but right now, right in the present, you get this one chance to live. Time and tide stop for no man. Either you're going to live life or not! I had to stop procrastinating and finally just start.

You can start changing right now. This moment. Today. Not tomorrow. Not next week. You can start the change process right now.

Denial.

If an obese or overweight person was telling me that they're happy and they're fine, I'd have to call them out on that. I have to say, "You're lying to yourself."

There's no way! There's not a chance. Don't kid yourself. Your life is not what you want it to be, but you CAN change. It's not hopeless. You're not fine. Be honest with yourself and make the change.

Selfishness

Let me unpack this one a little because although I've mentioned it a bit, I haven't dug into this topic fully. Most books don't. Nobody wants to hear about being selfish. When I could be honest that selfishness was the root of my problem, when I got honest about it, that's when it started to turn around for me.

When it comes down to it, selfishness is the root of almost every issue on the planet. Primarily it's not a just a political, economic or societal issue that's plaguing the world — those are just manifestations of the root problem — selfishness. Let me approach this topic again, without being preachy, from a faith perspective.

There's not a lot of answers in the bible that tell us *why* Jesus died. Paul, the Apostle mentioned that Jesus died for everyone, so that everyone, those who live, should no longer live for themselves, but for Him. (St. Paul - II Cor. 5:15). Essentially he's saying that Jesus died so that we wouldn't have to be selfish any longer. That's a game-changer!

I think if you look at what Jesus' life was about, it was always about giving. He gave up so much, he came down to earth to give to everybody else and a lot of times it was to give and to love even to people that hated him. No matter what he gave, no matter what he did, it was never good enough, but he still gave everything for others and he gave sacrificially.

I think that can be a huge lesson today because as a society, it seems the only people we care about is ourselves. The only time I might give to others is if it make me feel good, giving with a kickback. What's in it for me? Even our "sacrificial giving" can be selfish. How warped is that?

I think if people are really looking for true happiness, we need to consider Jesus' example and give to others selflessly, like He gave. I think if we give to others selflessly, that puts a stop to selfishness, one selfless act at a time. Stopping the selfishness inside of me was the beginning of the end of my problem. I just wanted to constantly eat what felt good, what I enjoyed, "me, me, me." The end result of that was going nowhere, fast. It would have killed me.

When I woke up and saw the empty seat beside me that my selfish, overweight self was taking from some one else, that's when I had enough and heard, "enough," bouncing around my head continually. That change from the inside out, for me, was a Divine moment. It was when something, Someone bigger than me, a Purpose, an Eternal Force, a Power within me, came along side of that word, that thought, "enough," and empowered me to change. Thanks for praying Mom! I know that Power was God's strength and love helping me.

I was invited recently to an interview where the host was asking about my weight gain. I told him that it was nobody's fault but my own and I was basically being selfish. I told him that I had nobody to blame but myself.

He said to me, "Tony, aren't you being a bit hard on yourself?"

I said, "No, not at all." It seems to me, that no one wants to accept responsibility for their own actions.

We have to.

With all my weight gain nobody forced me to eat what I ate. I'm not stupid. I'm not paralyzed. Nobody is putting a spoon up to my mouth and force-feeding me. I knew what I was doing. There was no problem or anything wrong with my body that was causing me to be that big. My issue was putting junk in my body continually, huge unaccountable excess, day in, day out. I'd eat chips and chocolate bars and ice cream in extreme quantities every day. Of course I was going to develop that body type that eventually looks like a tub of ice cream. There's no way around it.

For some reason now, we don't want to accept any responsibility for any bad things that happen to us in life. We blame it on the past, or our parents, or conservatives, or liberals, or the big banks, or corporations or a million other excuses. For me, in my case, the only way I got to be that size was just laziness and selfishness. It was about poor choices I made to affect other people. I showed a lack of respect for my own body; it was horrible what I did to myself.

That was the bottom line for me. It was nobody's fault but my own, but with God's help, I worked hard and it turned around. It's probably the hardest thing I've ever done. I just said, "enough!" I stopped eating junk and started walking. That was it!

Where Do I Start?

If you don't know where to start, or when to start, just start. Don't wait until tomorrow. Waiting until tomorrow or after the weekend or next week or after the next holiday or birthday or long weekend, that's how I put on all the weight.

Start right now. Seriously. You can do it.

Don't eat any more crap today and go for a walk. If I can go for a walk in Fort McMurray any day of the year where it gets to thirty-five degrees below zero (it doesn't matter if it's Celsius or Fahrenheit - either way, it's really cold) you can do it where you live too. I started walking when it was over 30 degrees Celsius with 330 extra pounds. You can do this. I did.

I believe in you. You're not alone.

Coaching Questions

Here are a few questions that you can consider to help you on your journey of lifestyle wellness. I don't really have a lot of answers, but hopefully these questions can help you honestly evaluate your situation and start planning your next courageous steps.

Questions:

Priorities?
What are my priorities in life?
What are my priorities with food?
Healthy food: when and what?
Junk food: how little? When?
What priorities am I missing out on because of bad habits?
What are my top priorities for the coming months and years?
How do I need to change my life's structure to accommodate these priorities?
Who should I speak with to help me realign these priorities who will then keep me on task?

Have I tried and failed many times?

If I'm stuck, whether it's 300 pounds I need to lose, or thirty pounds or three pounds…am I addicted to something?

Do I feel I need treats, or cheat days?

How can I change that thinking?

Do I look to food for comfort?

Who can help me change this thinking?

Accountability?

Are there people in my life that can ask me hard questions without me storming off in a temper tantrum or sulking?

Am I surrounded by honest community, people who can see through my smokescreens and call me on it?

Who are those people?

How can I be more intentional to embrace supportive community?

How often could we check in with each other realistically?

Selfishness?

Am I courageous enough to say *no* to myself?

Do I have the inner strength I need independent of others?

Am I courageous enough to ask for help?

Am I open to seeking God's help, or the help of a higher power like the 12-step program talks about?

What can I do to be more mindful of others?

How can I make the world a better place for 2 or 3 other people this week or this month?

Goals?

What measurable goals am I willing to set for eating?

For walking?

When will I start?

Who can I be accountable to with these goals?

How often do I need to re-evaluate these goals?

Commitment?

Am I ready to commit to starting a lifestyle change right now?

On a scale of 1-10 (where 10 is most) how committed am I to lifestyle change?

What would it take to make that commitment level an 8, 9 or 10?

What prevents me from starting with lifestyle change?

How can I change that immediately?

Who can help me follow through with these commitments?

About the Co-Author

Mark Griffin is a Ghostwriter based out of Ontario, Canada. This is Mark's sixth book, but first public by-line. Mark has written hundreds of scripts for television and prepared over five thousand presentations in his career as a communicator and author.

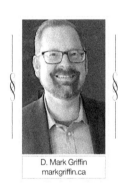

D. Mark Griffin
markgriffin.ca

▐▌ facebook.com/DeclaringLife

🐦 twitter.com/DMarkGriffin

📷 instagram.com/griff7mark